HELLO, BICYCLE

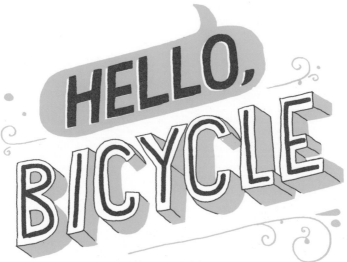

HELLO, BICYCLE

AN INSPIRED GUIDE TO THE TWO-WHEELED LIFE

ANNA BRONES

Illustrations by James Gulliver Hancock

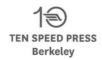

TEN SPEED PRESS
Berkeley

CONTENTS

INTRODUCTION

Two wheels. A bicycle isn't much more complicated than that.

In its simplest form, the bicycle is made up of two wheels, a frame, a chain, pedals, handlebars, and a seat. It is the most beautiful of machines, as aesthetically pleasing as it is functional. Today's bicycle isn't too far from its first incarnation in the early 1800s. Certainly, the bicycle has evolved, but ultimately its basic form has held up, and it is this lack of changes that speak to the bicycle's one true power: its simplicity.

One of humankind's greatest inventions was the wheel. The wheel was revolutionary; it changed everything—how we work, how we travel, how we live. Over the centuries, the wheel has been used in many machines and contraptions, but its basic form and function haven't changed at all. And wheels—two of them, to be precise—are exactly what make a bicycle so incredible. It's thanks to those two wheels, in line, that the bicycle is such a simple wonder. Just like the wheel, the bicycle, too, is revolutionary.

The bicycle is a simple mode of transportation, a simple way to transport cargo, a simple way to get out and exercise. You don't need any type of fuel except your own two legs to power a bicycle forward. Bike maintenance doesn't require a computer; a few tools and a little elbow grease will get you far. The bicycle is simply fun.

In a day and age where we are looking for ways to live more sustainable lives, build better communities, and be healthier, the bicycle has emerged as one of the best ways to achieve all three. If we have begun to embrace the bicycle with renewed interest, it's because the bicycle is in many ways the easiest solution to a multitude of problems. It won't fix every problem out there, but it's a good start—one that individuals, urban planners, and politicians are seeing as a meaningful tool to create positive change.

Why embrace a life on two wheels? Because above all, a life on two wheels is a simple life. It's about slowing down. It's about enjoying our surroundings. It's about finding beauty in the everyday. It's about going on rides with friends. It's about finding and building community. It's about feeling the wind on your face as you charge down a hill. It's about the feeling of pushing one foot down and then the other, that rhythmic meditation that is so enthralling and addicting. It's difficult to ride a bicycle without smiling. Bicycling feels good, and in our hectic, fast-paced modern lives, we need this.

But despite the bicycle's simplicity, the world of cycling can easily feel intimidating. If we haven't ridden one for some time (for *quite* some time), we don't know where to begin; we feel overwhelmed by all the things we think we are supposed to know. But here's the thing: it's the overcomplication of something simple that makes it intimidating. Want to get back to that exhilarating feeling of being a kid on a bicycle? All you need to do is strip away all of those overcomplications.

That's what this book is for. This book is for those of you who remember the excitement of getting your first bicycle. It's for those of you looking at those bike commuters on your way to work and wondering if you could do it, too. It's for anyone who ogles the bike parked at the store with a basket for groceries positioned on the front. This book is also for those of you who already ride but want to do a little more—

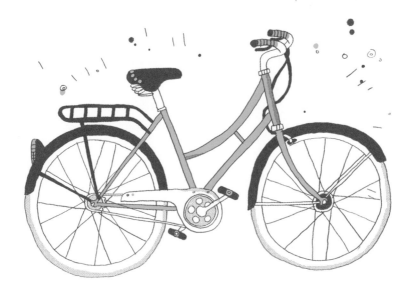

change your own tires, plan a cycling tour, or even find the inspiration to launch a pedal-powered business. It's for anyone who has ever said to themselves, "I want to ride more, but . . ."

It doesn't matter what comes after the "but." What matters is that you want to ride. That you are excited about the mere prospect of getting on a bicycle.

I think about the "why" of cycling a lot. As someone who often rides in an urban environment—dodging buses, ringing the bell at unaware pedestrians, internally cursing the lack of bike lanes—I can't help but look at myself and my fellow everyday cycling friends and wonder why we do it. Why throw ourselves into the middle of traffic, when we are so much less protected than if we were in a car? Why put up with buses and taxis and motorcycles, whose drivers seem as if they couldn't care less that a bicycle is on the road with them? The rational person would look at the intensity of cycling in some urban areas and think, "What on earth is wrong with these people?" Why do we ride? Because we love it. I could say that it's because I want to make a positive impact on my community, or it saves me money, or it gives me exercise. These are all excellent effects of cycling. But ultimately, if I peel back all the layers, it's an activity that I do simply because it makes me happy. I love to be on a bicycle.

Of course, love can often be undermined by fear. Not all of us live in bike-friendly communities, and for some people, deciding to ride a bicycle isn't an easy choice. It's an act that takes a lot of work. That being said, many of us live in places where we *could* ride more. I think part of the reason that we don't ride is fear—fear of traffic, of the lack of bike paths, of the limited amount of shoulder space to ride on, and so on. But I also think that it's partly because we haven't had the opportunity to reignite our love for cycling. Because there are a lot of cyclists out there who *do* put up with all of this scary stuff. All that hard stuff that should put them off cycling. But they ride anyway. Why? Because at the end of the day, they just want to be on their bicycles.

Someone recently told me about her trip to Amsterdam, where she spent the week on rented bicycles with her kids. "I always liked bikes, I own a bike, but it wasn't until I spent a week riding one in an urban setting where the bike rider rules the road that I fell in love." As an urban cyclist, I would love to live in Amsterdam, where bikes aren't just a mode of transportation, but a way of life. But I don't live in Amsterdam. Most of us don't. We have to learn from bike-friendly capitals like

Amsterdam and Copenhagen so that we can start pushing for those same policies that encourage people to get on bikes in our own communities. How do we start doing that? First and foremost, we begin with rediscovering the love of two wheels.

The point here is to get back to that initial love. That simplicity. Find it and you'll never look back.

The world of cycling is open to anyone who wants in. This book is here to help facilitate that process. It isn't a technical guide or a book about how to train for a race. It is a book inspired by a love for cycling, and by a desire to see more people in the world doing it. It is a book for inspiring you to do more by bicycle.

Where to begin? Maybe you're wondering about what kind of bike to buy, or what gear you need in order to bike commute, or how to take things to the next level and plan a bike trip. Whatever you are searching for, this book is here to ensure a smooth transition to a two-wheeled life. It's about embracing cycling, not just as a sport but also as a lifestyle. It's about slowing down and living intentionally. It's about celebrating, packing up a picnic and biking to your favorite park, throwing on your rain wear and pedaling off into the nastiest of winter storms. This book is about cycling, 365 days a year. And even if you miss a few, I want to make sure that you're looking forward to the next time you take your bicycle out for a spin.

People often say that bikes have the power to change the world. I definitely believe that they do. Why? Because they're simple. Because cycling is easy to learn. Because bikes are found around the world. But most important, again, because cycling makes us smile. It makes us feel great—and when something makes us feel great, we want to keep doing it again and again and again.

Let's fall back in love. Let's start pedaling.

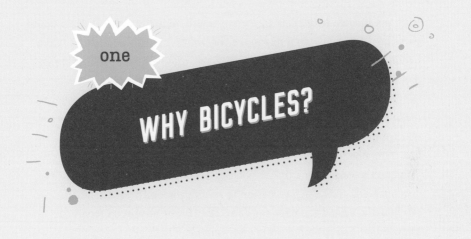

one

WHY BICYCLES?

If someone told you that there was one thing that you could do every single day that would make you healthier, help the environment, boost the economy, and maybe even make the world a better place, would you do it?

Well, good news! There is one thing you can do that accomplishes all of that: riding a bicycle.

THE MANY BENEFITS OF BICYCLES

Riding a bicycle may seem like just a small, unimportant act. How could pedaling once or twice a day make the world a better place? But while cycling is certainly a simple act—you are, after all, just pushing down one foot after the other—the benefits are limitless.

Bicycles make us smile, they keep us in good shape, and they help us make positive changes. Riding a bicycle is empowering, freeing, because you are dependent only on yourself. A bicycle gives you autonomy. The one thing needed to get you from point A to point B on a bicycle is *you*. You don't need to buy a ticket; you don't have to follow a timetable. You don't need to go to the gas station to refuel; you don't need to check the oil. You don't need special gear or vocabulary or advanced technical knowledge. You need a bicycle and yourself. That's all.

People who cycle regularly have been shown to be healthier and live longer, with better blood pressure and a lower likelihood of being overweight than their car-driving counterparts. Women who bike thirty minutes a day or more have a lower risk of breast cancer, and adolescents who bike are almost 50 percent less likely to be overweight as adults.

But the benefits of cycling aren't just personal. When we ride, we inherently make our communities a better place to live.

More cyclists on the road—who might otherwise be driving a car or taking the bus—means reduced carbon emissions. For example, in the bike-friendly Danish capital of Copenhagen, bike traffic prevents 90,000 tons of CO_2 from being emitted annually. If in the United States each of us made just one four-mile round-trip by bicycle instead of by car each week, we would burn almost two billion fewer gallons of gas per year. And you know what else that accomplishes? It helps reduce economic dependence on foreign oil. Cycling is patriotic!

How often does something that makes us feel personally great also offer an extensive list of external benefits? Even those riding a bicycle for only selfish reasons are doing their part (even if they don't realize it), benefiting the entire community around them.

Given all the benefits, what's stopping us from riding?

Many of us learned to ride as children, yet somewhere in the journey into adulthood we lose the art of cycling. Pull up a memory of your first bicycle. Maybe it was red, maybe it was blue. Maybe it had streamers on the handlebars. Maybe it had those crazy colored spoke beads that made noise as the wheels turned. Whatever your first bicycle looked like, chances are you probably remember it clearly. That first bicycle is

What Biking Won't Do to You

GIVE YOU "BIKE FACE"

In the late nineteenth century, female cyclists were warned that riding could lead to "bicycle face," a look of being exhausted and weary. In truth, if cycling gives you any kind of a face, it's a face with a smile!

TURN YOU INTO A CYCLING GEEK

Well, unless of course you want to be one. You can make cycling a part of your everyday life and stay perfectly normal—although eventually your two-wheeled life will become your new normal, which in turn might turn you into a *little* bit of a cycling geek. But that's not a bad thing.

FORCE YOU TO WEAR SPANDEX

You can ride in your everyday, normal clothes and feel good about it. No need to be intimidated because you don't have the "right" clothes. Eventually, if you start doing long road rides or racing, you might want sportier attire that's more comfortable for long stretches of cycling, but don't let a lack of special clothing get between you and your bicycle.

an inerasable vision forever etched into our memory. Remember learning how to ride that bicycle? Think back. You feel your father's, your mother's, your uncle's, your older sister's hand holding the back of the seat as they run beside you, making sure you don't fall. At first, you're timid. You pedal, reassured that someone is there to hold you. You get into a rhythm. You look to your side; whoever was holding you is gone. You are pedaling on your own. The exhilaration mounts. You are riding by yourself!

That first bicycle, and the process of learning how to ride, sticks with us for as long as we live, because our first bicycle represents our first taste of true freedom. The bicycle is a door to many opportunities, particularly for a child. It's a new, efficient mode of transportation, and one that you—and only you—are responsible for. Those first few pedal strokes without an adult holding on to the back of the bicycle to steady you are freeing. You are alive. You are in control. You can do anything.

Remember what it felt like to ride a bike as a child? It was fun. It was simple. If you wanted to hop on your bike, you didn't spend too long thinking about it; you just did it. It was freeing. You could go where you wanted. You could explore. You went fast. Really fast. You probably scraped your knees in a few tumbles, but you didn't care. You got back on the bicycle and did it all over again.

If we were once so in love with riding our bicycles, what is it that stops so many of us from doing it as we get older? Because we forget the bicycle's simplicity. Unfortunately, the bicycle's simplicity and pace are rarely accommodated in the design of urban and suburban sprawl. If there are bike lanes, there are few of them, and the built environment around us encourages four wheels and not two. But we also complicate the act of riding a bicycle, and in the face of those complications, many of us become intimidated.

25 Reasons Why You Should Ride a Bicycle

1. You will be healthier.

2. People will find you more attractive.

3. You can eat more and feel perfectly fine about it.

4. You'll make new friends.

5. It's budget friendly.

6. Your friends will admire your toned calves.

7. You don't need a parking space.

8. You can fit exercise into your everyday routine without even thinking about it.

9. A beer tastes better after a bike ride.

10. So does coffee.

11. Paying for a bike tune-up is much less expensive than buying gas on a regular basis.

12. You spend more time outside— something your mother was always telling you to do.

13. People have more respect for you when you show up to a dinner party having transported a cake on a two-wheeled vehicle.

14. Cycling is a stress reliever and emotional booster that doesn't require medication.

15. You'll never have to sit in rush-hour traffic.

16. Bike storage can also look like a really fancy interior design element in your house or apartment.

17. Riding in the rain is actually awesome.

18. Getting muddy is too.

19. You don't have to listen to boring talk radio during your commute.

20. Picnics are better by bicycle.

21. Bicycles are beautiful, even sexy.

22. Groceries look better in a bike basket.

23. Even five bikes still won't take up as much space as a car.

24. You'll have a new way to explore places when you travel.

25. You can name your bicycle and talk about it like it's a person.

If it's not the thought of riding in traffic that scares us, it may be the thought of going into a bicycle shop and not knowing what to ask for. Or it's thinking that we don't have the right clothes. Or we don't have a bicycle at all, and how do we even begin looking for one?

There is no reason to be afraid or intimidated; just about anyone who can walk can ride. And the more people who ride, the easier it becomes for even more people to do it. If we want to build a society that's more bike friendly, the best thing that we can do is to start cycling ourselves. Then we can get a friend cycling. And then another, and another.

This has already started to happen, and in many cities around the world, bike usage is growing, which benefits all of us.

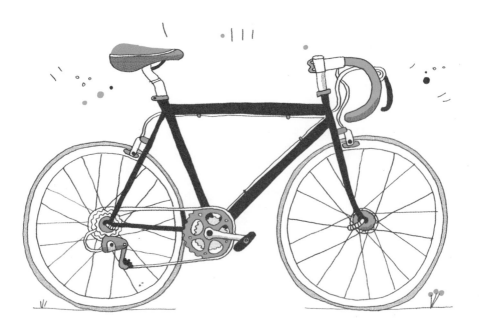

THE HISTORY OF THE BICYCLE

This current rise in the popularity of the bicycle—infiltrating all parts of pop culture, marketing campaigns, window displays, and fashion—might seem like a modern phenomenon, but this isn't cycling's first heyday.

While there were different human-powered wheeled vehicles designed before it, the first iteration of the bicycle as we know it came along in the early 1800s when a German, Karl Drais, released his "running machine," called the *draisienne*. This two-wheeled, steerable device was created as an alternative to transportation on horseback, garnering it the names "hobby horse" and "dandy horse." There were no gears or pedals, and riders pushed the vehicle forward with their own two feet on the ground, similar to today's balance bikes for children. A few years later, Denis Johnson of England designed a new and improved model, marketed to London aristocrats. It took London by storm. Tallyho!

In the 1860s, the velocipede was developed: a wooden contraption with two pedals attached to the front wheel and a fixed gear system, propelled like a tricycle. There is disagreement as to the original designer of the velocipede, but it was a Frenchman who made the first truly popular and commercialized design. A blacksmith who usually made carriage parts, Pierre Michaux, began making a version of the hobby horse with pedals in 1867, with the help of two wealthy Parisian brothers, Aimé and René Olivier. Another Frenchman, Pierre Lallement, is also credited with being one of the first to attach pedals to the front wheel, and in 1866 he filed the first bicycle patent with the U.S. patent office.

However, this velocipede was hard to ride, and in England it got the name "bone shaker" for its rough effects on the rider. In search of a ride that went faster, manufacturers began making the front wheel much larger, leading to the contraption known as the "penny-farthing"

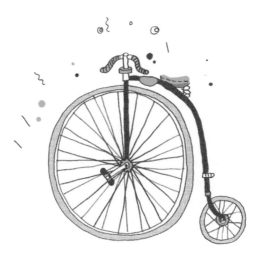

(also known as the "high wheeler"). Challenging to ride, penny-farthings didn't last long, as riders and manufacturers sought out safer devices, but the allure of these vehicles has carried over into modern times, and those attracted to the thrill of these high-wheeled bicycles can still find them today.

An Englishman was the one to come up with the solution to the safety challenges of the high wheelers. In 1884, John Kemp Starley introduced his Rover safety bicycle, which was safe in comparison to the high wheelers of the time. Because of this design, Starley is widely considered the inventor of the modern bicycle.

Bike culture quickly spread across Europe and the United States, and toward the end of the nineteenth century cycling was all the rage. By one estimate, in 1897 two million bicycles were manufactured in the United States, about one bicycle for every thirty people at the time. Why were people embracing bicycles? Because they gave them freedom. This was the age of the horse and buggy, a method of transportation that was not within everyone's budget. In this period, bicycles also became a critical part of the women's suffrage movement, since bicycles were a vehicle to freedom and independence.

Today cycling is once again gaining momentum. According to the U.S. Census Bureau, from 2000 to 2012, the number of U.S. bicycle commuters increased by 60 percent. Americans spend $81 billion on biking annually; the industry that meets this demand is responsible for over 770,000 jobs. Rediscovering our love for bicycles is having a positive effect.

Important Dates in Bike History

1891 → Bike polo first appears in Ireland, a "polo on wheels" instead of horses.

1894 → The first bamboo bikes are manufactured.

1895 → Annie Londonberry becomes the first woman to cycle around the world, with the help of trains and ships—a trip that takes fifteen months.

1896 → Five track events and a road race are part of the first modern Olympic Games.

1896 → Susan B. Anthony declares that the bicycle "has done more to emancipate women than anything else in the world."

1897 → The 25th Infantry Buffalo Soldiers ride 1,900 miles from Missoula, Montana, to Saint Louis, Missouri.

1899 → Charles Murphy becomes the first man to ride a bike at sixty miles per hour.

1903 → The first Tour de France race is held.

1958 → The first ever bicycling World Championship for women is held in Reims, France.

1963 → Schwinn introduces the Stingray, its first banana seat bike.

1970s → In Marin County, California, a group of cyclists starts adapting vintage clunker bikes to ride downhill. Mountain biking is born.

1986 → Greg LeMond is the first American to win the Tour de France.

1993 → First bicycle messenger championships held in Berlin, Germany.

1996 → Mountain biking becomes an official Olympic sport.

2005 → Lance Armstrong wins his seventh consecutive Tour de France title, of which he is later stripped because of his use of performance-enhancing drugs.

2014 → The inaugural edition of La Course, a one-day women's race held on the final day of the Tour de France (which is not open to women cyclists).

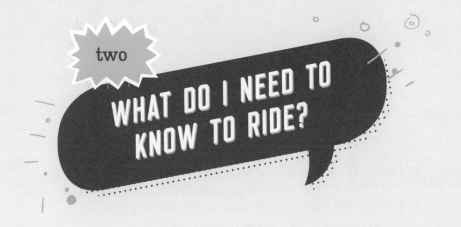

two

WHAT DO I NEED TO KNOW TO RIDE?

Now that you've decided that you want to make cycling a part of your life, what do you need to know? Should you buy a new bike or a used one? How should you store your bike? What if you get in a bike accident? There are a lot of questions when it comes to jumping into the world of cycling, but there's no need to feel intimidated. This chapter looks at some of the most basic questions related to the essentials you need to make riding a seamless part of your life.

WHAT KIND OF A BICYCLE DO I NEED?

When you've decided that you want to make biking a part of your everyday lifestyle, the next important question is this: what kind of bicycle is best for you?

There are, of course, many types of bicycles out there, and it all depends on what you're planning to do with your two-wheeled steed. A bicycle used for long weekend rides could be very different from one used for occasional grocery runs. Certainly, this is not an argument for buying a bicycle for every distinctive use (although if you get bitten by the biking bug and want to use it like that, feel free), but simply a reminder that you need to determine what you're looking for. Give some thought to what you are going to use your bicycle for the most. There's no point in buying a bicycle that doesn't fit your needs and then ends up sitting in the garage.

Let's start with the basics: you do not need a fancy bicycle.

While bicycles are undeniably beautiful, you don't get one for its looks; you get it for riding. And though an expensive, beautifully painted, well-tuned bicycle is certainly alluring, there's something to be said for the old beater ten-speed that has been sitting in someone's garage for fifteen years. It just may take a little extra work to get it back up and running.

To assess which bike is right for you, start with these two essential questions:

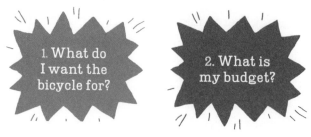

1. What do I want the bicycle for?

2. What is my budget?

What do I want the bicycle for?

To determine what type of bicycle you want to buy, you have to assess your main use of the bicycle. Are you wanting to go explore dirt trails on the weekend, or are you looking for a bike that you can pedal to work every day? What the bicycle will be used for will change what you look for when you are bicycle shopping.

Sport → You want to get out and ride on the weekends, preferably fast and hard.

Fun → You want to take part in local community rides and hop on the bicycle when the mood strikes you, not necessarily with a destination in mind, but just to get out and feel the air on your face for a bit.

Commuting → You're looking to drive your car a little less and are hoping to ride to work a few days a week.

Transport and cargo → You want the two-wheeled minivan—the cargo bike that holds the entire family *and* the dog. You're planning on grocery shopping by bike and potentially giving up the car entirely.

All of the above → You just want to ride, be it for work or to grocery shop. Oh, and if you could get in a long weekend ride on the same bike, that would be great, too.

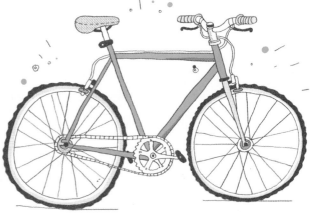

If you're getting your first bicycle, you will probably want to consider one that can serve a variety of purposes. This means that if you think you may want to go on some longer weekend rides, you probably don't want a beach cruiser. And if you're planning on using your bicycle mostly for commuting to work, you probably don't need a mountain bike with shock suspension—unless, of course, your office can be reached via a long single track trail (and if it is, I commend your choice of office). Most likely, you'll want a bicycle that has a few gears, is comfortable to ride, and isn't too expensive.

What is my budget?

Setting a budget is an essential part of buying a bicycle, because it will guide your buying decisions. The good part is that there are always options no matter what the budget. Factor in that if you don't already own essential bike accessories like lights, lock, and a helmet; those must be a part of your budget as well. You may choose to buy a very simple used model and get some work done to it. Or you may choose to buy a new bicycle that is entirely kitted out from the get-go. If you are planning to use your bike every day, then your bicycle isn't just an accessory, it's your main mode of transportation and therefore a necessity. This can easily justify a bigger budget. A bicycle that's just going to be for a ride here and there, however, might necessitate a smaller percentage of your overall household budget. Here you can put it in the same category as your budget for other fun things, like sports equipment and entertainment.

BUYING YOUR BICYCLE

Once you've established what you want the bike for and how much you can spend, the shopping fun begins. Even if you're set on a certain type of bicycle, it's always good to test a variety of models to see how they all feel and handle. You may think you're in the market for a cargo bike, but maybe a simple single speed with a big basket in front will work. Regardless of whether you buy new or used, once you've identified what you need the bicycle for, buying it is about trying to get to know as much as you can about your options before you buy.

Going to the bike shop to do a test ride is like going on a first date: you'll need to pedal a bike around the block a few times before you commit. Don't be afraid to go back for a second, third, and fourth date before making a full commitment. There's no point in jumping into a relationship with a bicycle that you don't really like!

Buying a used bicycle

Go ahead, drool over all those shiny new bikes in the bike store, even if you don't have the budget for them. But while new bikes are glorious and finely tuned, used ones can be just as good and sometimes are even better. They come with a story, after all. Here's another consideration: while a beautiful, sleek, new bicycle with all of the bells and whistles may be tempting, once you buy it, you're going to feel a certain obligation to keep it clean and in tip-top shape. This can mean that sometimes with a new bicycle you'll be afraid to get it dirty or to knock it up a bit. You'll dodge puddles so as not to get the fenders muddy. You won't lock it up on the street, for fear of scuffing it (and then—oh no!—good-bye, Gorgeous). While a bicycle is meant to be taken care of, an everyday bicycle is meant to be used, and often. You want a workhorse, and spending less on a used bicycle may help you to feel less afraid of getting it a little roughed up. That's a good thing.

WHERE TO BUY USED

Your city may have stores that specialize in used bike sales; if not, the Internet abounds with people looking to make a little cash off of the two wheels that they aren't using anymore. Garage sales can also be the place for great bike finds, and if you live in a city with an active bike community, there may be special bike sale events; local bike organizations are a great resource for finding these. Sometimes bike shops will also do sales specializing in used bicycles. As with buying any secondhand item, if you're in the market for a used bicycle, remember that it may take some time to find the right one. Keep your eyes and ears open, explore your options, and eventually you'll end up with the bicycle love of your life.

WHAT TO LOOK FOR IN A USED BIKE

The one caveat with buying used is that you need to be able to give the bike a thorough inspection to determine what mechanical shape it is in. Above all, if you're buying a used bike you want to ask questions about its former life. You want to ask a lot of questions up front to see whether the bike is going to stick around or whether you should move on immediately. How much did the previous user ride it? Where did they ride it? Did they do regular maintenance on the bicycle? Did they replace any parts? A used bike with a lot of love put into it can be just as good as a new bicycle—and way friendlier on the wallet, leaving you extra money for accessories. Fortunately, a bicycle isn't as complicated and inscrutable as a car, and even the beginner cyclist can assess whether or not a bicycle is in good working order. Tires and seats can be changed, but you want to ensure that the essential parts, like the frame, are solid and functional. Not sure if you are up to the task yourself? Ask around; someone in your circle of friends and friends of friends is probably a budding bike geek and may be better versed than you are in the technicalities of the bicycle. Take them along and have them help with a once-over of the bike to determine exactly what shape it's in, or refer to the following tips.

David Brumsickle, owner of Silverdale Cyclery in Silverdale, Washington, has seen a lot of bicycles in his career. He started his bike shop in 1985, and he's been helping people fall in love with cycling ever since. Here are his tips for what to look for in a potential used bike.

Make certain that the bike is a reasonably good fit. A bike that fits well usually allows you to stand over the frame with just a bit of clearance. It will allow you to raise or lower the saddle enough that your knee is nearly straightened out when you press a pedal all the way down. You should also be able to reach a spot on the handlebars where you can comfortably operate the brakes and shifters without locking your elbows. If a bike is too big, it will be awkward to get on and off. It will also feel too long between seat and bars, forcing you to lean too far forward. If it's too small, you may not be able to raise the seat enough for your height and you will be uncomfortable pedaling.

Make sure that the wheels aren't damaged. This can be really expensive to fix and can easily be a deal breaker. Spin them and watch them rotate. Look at the gap between the brake pads and the rim of the wheel. The wheel should rotate in a straight path without obvious wobbling. Also look for dents in the rim. These are almost impossible to fix and can

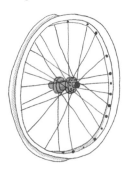

affect your ability to stop. Look and feel for a smooth braking surface without spots the brakes can catch on. Also note that chromed steel rims often appear on older bikes. These wheels are much heavier than aluminum ones and are rarely found on modern bicycles. These rims offer inferior stopping power and dent easily, so they are best avoided, or replaced if your bike comes with them. Tires can easily be replaced, but replacing an entire wheel is much more expensive, so make sure that the wheels are in good condition.

Make sure that the frame is not bent or cracked. This also can be a deal breaker. Look closely at the frame junction just behind the front brake. It shouldn't look wrinkled. Look carefully at the fork for signs of being bent backward. Give the frame a careful inspection for cracks, excessive rust, or major dents.

Look at the condition of the drivetrain. The drivetrain—that is, the chain, gears, and so on—is usually on the right side of the bicycle. When the bike is pedaled or rolled forward, the crank should rotate without an obvious wobble. If your potential bike has derailleurs (the system that allows you to change gears), you should be able to operate the shifters from the handlebars and at least see the derailleurs move a little.

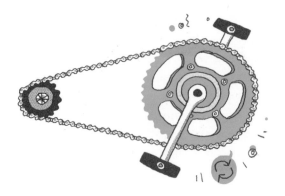

HELLO, BICYCLE

Check the brakes. You should be able to squeeze the brake levers and feel the brakes stop the bike as you roll it forward.

Rust isn't necessarily a deal breaker. Many rusty or broken parts can be replaced inexpensively by someone with a mechanical bent. A fine example is a rusty chain. Sometimes nice bikes get abandoned because they've been left outside and the chain is rusty. A new chain and some oil can bring these back to life in a few minutes.

Buying a new bicycle

There are a few undeniable advantages to buying a new bicycle rather than a used one. The first, of course, is that there is no wear or damage. Second, whereas a used bicycle may need a little work to bring it back to life, a new bicycle can be ridden straight out of the shop, and when you do, it is going to get a lot of compliments. (Don't be surprised when your new bicycle gets hit on.)

Investing in a new bicycle is similar to investing in a new car or computer; you'll have a warranty on parts and the frame, and there may even be some type of free service agreement. You're not only buying a new bicycle; you're also ensuring that it's going to get taken care of if something goes wrong.

You don't always have to pay the full list price for a new bicycle. Ask your local bike shop about sales. Since new models come out every year, if you're willing to buy at a certain time of year, there are always deals to be had. Of course, you can always walk right into a bike shop when the mood strikes you and buy a new bicycle. If you want to make a good investment, however, and not just a spur-of-the-moment purchase, buying a bicycle is about identifying all the things that you want from your ride (as we have already discussed), and then keeping an eye out so that when your ideal steed is offered at a good price, you can snap it up.

Whether you're buying new or used, remember this: you want a bicycle that isn't just an accessory; you want it to be a part of your everyday life. You want to feel great on it. Your bicycle is your new partner in crime; choose one that's going to have your back.

. . . .

MAKE YOUR BICYCLE *YOURS*

. . . .

Both brand-new and used bicycles can be a great starting point for customization. If you get a good deal on a basic model, you can deck it out yourself. Fancy fenders, a wine crate on the back for transporting groceries, and a new paint job can all make your bicycle your very own.

Should I get a custom-built bicycle?

The best bike out there for you is the one that you are going to be happy to ride. This means that when you're just starting out, it's perfectly fine to start with an inexpensive used bicycle. Two wheels is really all you need.

But eventually, as you do more and more bicycling, you may want to move into something a little nicer, something that is more customized to the kind of riding you are doing, or simply one that fits your size and personality a little better than what you can find on the regular bike market. This is where the custom-built bicycle comes in.

There are a variety of reasons to get a custom-built bicycle. Some people go custom because they want something that fits them perfectly, or because they want a bicycle that's finely tuned to the type of riding that they are doing. Others like the craftsmanship that goes into a custom bicycle, and the fact that they can ensure that the bicycle is produced more locally than other options, and by someone they can talk to, face to face. This makes the bike-purchasing process much more personal.

KNOW WHAT YOU'RE AFTER

Not everyone goes custom, of course, because these bicycles do come at a cost. The important thing to consider when going custom is that you need to be very clear about what you want. A bike builder is running a business, and while they are there to help you figure out what you need and to build the bicycle that is right for you, it's a much easier process if you know what you want going in. You don't want to be sending them an email every week with yet another thing that you thought of that you might need.

THE TIME AND MONEY OF CUSTOM BUILDING

If you're going to go custom, the two most important things to keep in mind are price and time. You need to budget for the bicycle you want; if you are already committed to getting a custom ride, this is not the time to be cutting corners. Investing in a custom bicycle is investing in a bicycle for life, so make sure you are getting what you want. Given all the work that goes into custom bike building, make sure that you are also being realistic about how long it's going to take to get your bicycle built. Don't expect to turn in your order and have your bicycle in a week. Some bike builders have very long wait times. But good things do come to those who wait, and that's certainly the case for a custom bicycle.

WHAT TO EXPECT WHEN YOU ARE GETTING A CUSTOM BICYCLE

Getting a custom bicycle is a much different process from just going to the bike shop and picking out a bicycle. Natalie Ramsland, who founded Sweetpea Bicycles in 2005, knows all about this process. At Sweetpea, Ramsland builds bikes that "will love you back," working with her clients to figure out the bicycle that will work best for them, and she knows all about what you should expect if you decide to get a custom-built bicycle.

Basic Bike Vocabulary

Jump into the cycling world, and you'll quickly encounter an entire language that at first just might sound a little foreign. There are many words and phrases specific to the bike world; here are a few to get you started.

CADENCE → This is the rhythm of your pedaling—in other words, the cycling pedaling rate, measured in revolutions per minute.

CENTURY → A hundred-mile ride.

CHAINRING TATTOO → When your calf rubs up against the bike chain and you get a nice (temporary) bike tattoo imprinted on your skin thanks to the grease.

CHAMOIS → The padding in cycling shorts (once made of leather chamois), which are not supposed to be worn with underwear.

CLIPLESS PEDALS → Ironically, these are actually the pedals that you clip cycling shoes into, and you need special shoes to do so.

CLUNKER → Also called a "beater bike," this is your bike that's well used and well loved, and maybe a little rough around the edges from all the use, but that you're happy to take out when you don't want to worry about its taking a beating.

CRIT → Abbreviation for "criterium," a short bike race held on city streets.

DOWNSHIFT → When you shift to a lower gear, which you do to make riding a bit easier, such as when you're going up a hill.

DRAFTING → When you ride behind another cyclist and, thanks to aerodynamics, get "pulled" along, saving some of your energy.

GRANNY GEAR → Slang for the lowest gear ratio possible.

KIT → Basically a bike outfit: matching jersey, shorts, jacket, sometimes even socks.

LSD → No, not that kind of LSD. This stands for *long slow distance* training—in other words, putting in your miles.

METRIC CENTURY → A ride that's one hundred kilometers (sixty-two miles) long.

PANNIERS → Those fancy bags, often used by bike tourers or commuters, that hang on the sides of the wheel, supported by a frame placed on either the front or back wheel, sometimes even both.

SADDLE → A bike seat.

TOE CLIPS → Metal or plastic baskets that are attached to your pedals, with a strap attachment that goes around your foot. Keeps your foot in place on the pedal and doesn't require special shoes.

UPSHIFT → When you shift to a higher gear because you are pedaling too fast and don't have any resistance.

You are worthy of a custom bike. No matter your riding ability, age, or self-proclaimed level of coolness, the only requirement for getting a custom bike should be your love of riding. Too many people delay or discount a custom bike because they don't feel [fill in the blank] enough. You, dear cyclist, are enough.

Prioritize bike fit. If your bike builder is taking only a few basic measurements from your body, you are getting a custom bike with an approximate size, not a truly custom fit. The fact that this is a common practice makes it no less of a tragedy! Find a bike fitter who can identify the proper riding position for your body, given all of its quirks and strengths. Your bike builder can then build you a bike that positively resonates with the energy you put into it.

Go ahead and get the fender mounts. At the outset, you may think that your current bike will become your rain bike and that your custom bike is destined to see only sunshine and tailwinds. But once you have a bike that fits you beautifully, you'll want to ride it all the time, even when it rains. And nothing can brighten up a dreary day like a ride on your beloved bike.

Keep 'em quiet in the cheap seats! Ramsland jokingly warns her customers that she assesses a Boyfriend Charge of $500 on any bike order for which there is a bike expert in the customer's life who is telling her what she wants—or ought to want. The best bike that she or any other builder can build is for the person who will be riding the bike. Tell those "bike experts" to go get their own awesome bike.

Touch-up paint is better than perfection. Don't let your bike become too precious in your mind. You should ride your bike with wild abandon, love every minute of it, and expect it to gather the patina of good, hard living. The touch-up paint is mostly to make you feel better—not to fix anything on the bicycle. You don't need to feel obligated to keep your bike looking like it just rolled off of the showroom floor.

STORING YOUR BICYCLE

Whether it's going to be inside or outside, how you store your bicycle is an important thing to consider, not only for the physical state of your bicycle but also for ensuring that it doesn't get stolen.

How to store your bicycle outside

No matter how well we lock up our bicycles, sometimes terrible things do happen. Knowing that there are bike thieves out there, here are some tips for some good habits to get into when locking up your bike, to ensure that you've done everything in your power to keep that bicycle safe.

CONSIDER YOUR SURROUNDINGS

Some areas are safer to park in than others: for example, a busy street with lots of people as opposed to a dark alleyway. Whenever you have a choice, always opt for the safer location. But remember this: those nasty bike thieves can be lurking anywhere. Don't make assumptions about what looks like a safe neighborhood. Always lock that bicycle up!

ALWAYS LOCK TO A SOLID, FIXED OBJECT

If there's not a designated bike parking structure, then find the next best thing. Look for a solid, fixed object that can't be moved or unbolted. It might seem obvious, but the point is to lock to something that isn't going to move. Street sign poles work great, as well as railings, as long as they are sturdy and well-bolted. Sometimes you just have to get creative.

THINK ABOUT THOSE WHEELS

Bike thieves will take what they can get. If your bicycle has quick-release wheels, then pay particular attention to those. For shorter stops, simply locking through the frame and front wheel may be enough For longer-term parking, you may want to consider using the cable and U-lock method (see page 33) to ensure that both wheels are secured.

The essentials of locking your bicycle

Some cyclists spend most of their time on road rides where they don't do much stopping between point A and point B. This type of riding may not necessitate a super vigilant approach to locking the bicycle, as you won't be stopping for long periods of time. But if you stop for a post-ride coffee at a café, be sure to sit outside with your bicycle. If, however, you're planning on using your bicycle for commuting or just getting around town, there's no denying that you need a lock. Unless you live in small-town bicycle utopia where people are kind enough to not steal bikes and you can leave it outside a shop unlocked and expect to find it when you return (these places do exist), a good lock is an absolute must.

WHAT LOCK SHOULD YOU GET?

Here's the thing about buying a lock: this is not the time to save money. While you can save a few bucks by buying a used bicycle or a bicycle that needs some work, when it comes to a lock, you want the best of the best. A lock isn't essential to keeping your bicycle functioning, but it's essential to keeping your bicycle—full stop.

Cable and chain locks come in many forms and lengths. Some have loops at the end, intended to be used with a padlock or U-lock (discussed next), and some come with their own locking system, like a combination lock. The benefit of a cable or chain lock is that, because they are flexible, you can lock your bike in a variety of situations. The drawback is that not all cables and chains are created equal, and if you buy one of lower quality, there's a chance that it could be cut and your bike stolen. Your local bike shop can recommend a good one.

A U-lock gets its name from its shape. A U-shaped section slips into a straight bar with a locking mechanism inside that you open and close with a key. U-locks provide greater security because they tend to be much harder to cut than chains or cables. The drawbacks of a U-lock are that they are heavy (that means they're not the ideal lock when you're on a long ride and just need to lock up to quickly run into a store to buy another granola bar) and, because they are rigid, they don't allow you to get creative with your locking method. This can prove problematic when you're in a place where there isn't a lot of bike parking and you're stuck locking your bike to a telephone pole or something of the like; a U-lock won't fit around it. But U-locks are, hands down, your best option for not getting your bike stolen—the Kryptonite brand's models even come with antitheft protection, in the event your lock doesn't do its job—and you can solve the rigidity problem by also carrying a cable (read on).

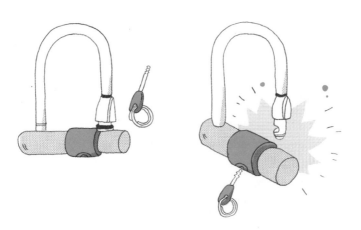

HOW TO LOCK

There are a few options for locking your bike, and what you do will depend on the surroundings (such as the safety level of neighborhood), how long you are locking the bike for, and your personal preference and risk/comfort level. Regardless of what you choose to do, always be sure to lock a fixed part of your bicycle (that is, the frame) to a fixed object. If you lock to just the wheel, without going through the frame, it's easy for someone to steal the frame. You may not want a bicycle without a front wheel, but bicycle thieves don't care one bit. They will take what they can get.

The best way to keep your bike safe is to double up, especially if you own a bike that makes other people drool. A U-lock and cable lock can be used together to make your locking system extra secure. The cable or chain can be run through the wheels and around the bike, then attached to the U-lock, which is locked to a fixed object, like the pole of a street sign or a designated bike parking structure.

- Detach the front wheel, place it next to the back wheel, and lock both wheels and the frame to a fixed structure. This is by far the safest option, particularly if your bicycle has quick-release wheels, but it's also the most time consuming. A good option if you need to leave your bicycle for an extended period of time.

- Lock the back wheel and frame to a fixed structure, and run a cable through the front wheel. This ensures that you have the frame and both wheels securely locked.

- Lock the back wheel and frame to a fixed structure. This will leave your front wheel unlocked, so this is a better option for bicycles with a fixed front wheel and not a quick release.

- Lock both the back wheel and the front wheel to a fixed structure with two different U-locks. If you carry two separate U-locks, then you can individually lock the front and back wheels.

- Lock the front wheel and the frame to a fixed structure. You will notice that a lot of people lock their bicycles this way, as it's simple and easy, particularly if they don't have quick-release wheels, as they are harder to remove.

CARRYING YOUR LOCKS

Since you never know when you're going to want to stop, always keep your bike lock with you. This, of course, presents the question of storage. Some U-locks come with a mount that can be attached to your bike to hold your U-lock while riding. You'll often see cable locks looped around handlebars or around the bicycle seat stem. There is also the backpack/purse method; this means carrying the extra weight on you as opposed to putting it on the bicycle, but it's always practical. If your bicycle is equipped with panniers, you can easily carry the lock(s) there. You can also wear a cable and U-lock around your body, like a messenger bag, for easy carrying.

Storing your bicycle inside

Locking up your bike temporarily when going into a grocery store or hanging out at a friend's house is one thing; more permanent bike storage is quite another. Where do you put your bicycle overnight?

We don't all have the luxury of living in a place with good bike parking. If that's the case for you, it's time to think seriously about your own setup. When an apartment building or workspace doesn't provide adequate outdoor bike parking, some people prefer to take their bicycle indoors. This keeps it more protected not only from bike theft but also from the elements; you don't want a nice bicycle sitting out in the rain day after day.

Bicycles get cranky when they're left outside and unattended; you want to be giving that bicycle some love. That means a nice dry space where the bicycle feels at home. Keep it out of the rain (and snow) if at all possible. There are different storage options for different living spaces. You may go to someone's house and see a bicycle parked in the entryway. Or even the kitchen. Besides simply propping the bicycle up against a wall, you can also install a bike storage system. An easy and budget-friendly option, if you have the space, is to screw a heavy-duty hook into a wall. On a wall with dry wall or plaster, be sure that you are drilling into a beam, easy to do by using a stud finder. You then lift the bike, hang the front wheel off of the hook, and let the back wheel rest on the wall, so that it looks like the bicycle is driving up the wall. For the more design savvy, you may want to consider a wall-hanging setup, which lets your bike double as an interior accent.

WHAT DO I DO IF MY BIKE IS STOLEN?

This is a situation that no cyclist would wish upon another, but unfortunately, it does happen. And often a stolen bicycle is a lost bicycle, which is why many cyclists choose to have a more inexpensive, older model for their everyday bicycle that they use around town. The loss of one of these is much less traumatic than the theft of a fancy road bike that you took out a small loan to buy.

Be prepared

Dealing with bike theft starts with prevention, and that means noting the serial number of your bicycle and keeping it in a safe spot that you can remember; you'll need it when you report your bike theft to the authorities. Keep photos of your bicycle as well; these will be much more helpful to the authorities than a description like "Um, well, it's red, with wheels." You can even add your information to one of several online bike databases like the National Bike Registry. These are maintained and used in conjunction with the authorities to ensure that bicycles are returned to their rightful owners.

Getting your bicycle back

Even if and when your bicycle is recovered by the authorities, the number of bicycles actually returned to their owners is unfortunately miniscule. The best thing that you can do is to file a police report right away. Better to report and not find your bicycle than to not report and wonder what might have happened if you had taken the time to go down to the station.

Besides reporting your stolen bicycle to the authorities, there are some other actions you can take. Check out online classified websites, like Craigslist, in your area for bicycles whose description matches your own. If you do happen to find your bike, alert the authorities. There are plenty of stories of people stealing their own bikes back, but don't put yourself in a dodgy situation; better to let the authorities handle it. Safety first!

Tell your friends, and share photos of your bicycle online; the more people in the bike community who know that your bike is missing and what it looks like, the greater the chance that someone might spot it. However, keep in mind that bike theft usually isn't the top priority for police departments, so you may just have to say your mental good-byes to your bicycle and go back to square one and get a new one.

BICYCLE ACCESSORIES

A bicycle isn't all that you need. Any everyday rider will know that there are a few essentials you can't live, or ride, without. Let's cover the basics.

Be seen

One bicycle accessory that you must not skimp on is a good light setup. A safe rider is a rider who is seen by others. This means a front light *and* a back light, and maybe even some spoke lights and reflective straps. Some states—California and Oregon, for example—even have light laws in place, requiring cyclists to have a white light in the front and a red reflector or light in the back.

Many lights come with a mount that attaches to your bike and stays on there permanently; then the light gets slipped on and off. When you go out for a night on the town, you can easily pull your light off where you park the bike, pop it in your bag, and ensure that it doesn't get stolen while you're off having a good time. No one wants to spend good money on a light only to have it disappear.

There are also clip-on lights, which are great if you're borrowing a bicycle and not sure about the light setup. These can be clipped to your clothes or bag or even a part of the bicycle. Even if you ride the same bicycle every day and have a good light setup, it's great to have one of these with you as a backup light in the event that one of your own lights fails.

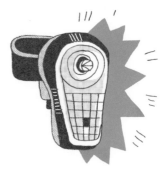

Lights aren't just for the dark of night. A foggy morning or rainy afternoon can definitely necessitate some extra visibility, and a light can provide just that. Flashing LED lights are also helpful, as they draw a motorist's attention to you, increasing the likelihood of being seen.

In addition to lights, reflective straps not only make a cyclist more visible, but they can also double to protect your pants from that dirty chain ring. Think of them as a current and bike-friendly version of the slap bracelet of the 1980s and 1990s.

Some regular commuters also believe in a high-visibility reflective vest, sort of like the ones you see construction workers wearing. A bright Day-Glo orange cyclist is hard to miss.

Be heard

Depending on where you live and do most of your riding, you may find that a bell or even a horn can be quite useful. That pedestrian who is unknowingly crossing the street without looking to see if a bike is barreling down on them? Much easier to ring a bell a few times than yell. Just like with a car, however, remember to be a cyclist who rings that bell respectfully and only when necessary.

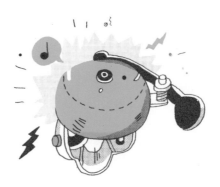

Protect your brain

While there are people who will argue for and against helmets, look at it this way: in a really bad accident, a helmet might not save you, but wouldn't you be happier wearing one in the event that it does? Let's put it another way: no one has ever said, "I wish I hadn't been wearing a helmet."

It's important to find a helmet that is comfortable and fits well, and while we all know that safety isn't about looks, if you buy one whose looks you don't really like, you won't want to wear it.

The other thing to consider is what kind of cycling you will be doing. Buy a helmet that suits your needs—if you are unsure of what you need, talk to a bike shop employee who can ensure that you buy a helmet that is the right size and fits you properly.

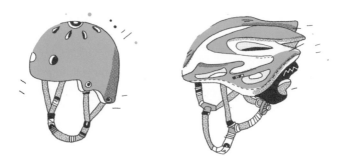

Sportier cycling helmets are great if you are planning on doing a lot of long rides or regular commuting, as they are ventilated, and there are some very lightweight versions. Some urban commuters prefer a helmet that looks a little less sporty, however; for them, there are the helmets that look a little more like a motorcycle helmet.

Carrying stuff on your bicycle

One of the bicycle accessories you may want to consider if you're using your bicycle for everyday use is some type of carrying device. Backpacks and messenger bags work great for carrying smaller, less heavy, and less bulky loads while cycling, but for heavier or bulkier items, you want the bicycle to carry it, not you. If you want to shift that weight and bulk off your body and onto the bicycle—and also keep the sweat off your back—you may be in the market for a basket.

Let's be honest: a basket on a bicycle looks damn good. It gets our inner European to light up. It also allows you to transport a variety of items—groceries, a six-pack of beer, a pile of books from the library—without having to worry about remembering to take a bag with you when you leave the house. Baskets come in all shapes, sizes, and materials. A wooden basket can be beautiful, but if you're riding in the rain 90 percent of the year, you may want something made from aluminum or stainless steel.

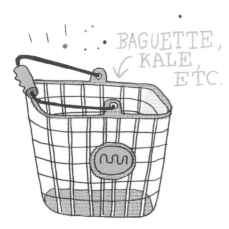

BAGUETTE, KALE, ETC.

Beyond baskets, you can also outfit your bicycle to accommodate a box or a crate. You don't have to buy one built specifically for your bike; many cyclists are happy to retrofit an old milk crate or produce box to be their carrying device. These can be used for both the front and the back of the bicycle, but regardless of where you are placing the basket, you will need a pannier rack to hold it.

HOW TO INSTALL A WOODEN CRATE

You will need: a wooden crate, a pannier rack (mounted on front or back of bicycle), 2 mending plates, a drill and drill bit the same diameter as the holes in your mending plates, 4 bolts, 4 nuts, 4 washers, a screwdriver, a wrench (adjustable or same size as nut), and 4 corner braces for the crate (optional). Note that the sizes of the mending plates, bolts, and corner braces will depend on the size and thickness of your crate. Be sure to measure before you buy.

To get your hands on a wooden wine or produce crate, check out vintage stores, yard sales, or ask a wine shop if they have any extras you can get your hands on. Before you start, make sure your crate is clean. Want to give your crate an extra kick? Go wild and paint. Remember that if you live in an area where rain is an issue, treating it so that it's waterproof will ensure that the crate has a long and healthy life. If you want a stronger crate, you can also reinforce the corners with corner braces.

Where you drill your holes will depend on the size of the crate and the dimensions of the pannier rack. Regardless of the size, you want to ensure that your mending plates will be evenly placed, and as far away from each other as possible, without going off the pannier rack, to ensure that the weight of the crate is evenly distributed. The middle of the crate should sit on top of the pannier rack.

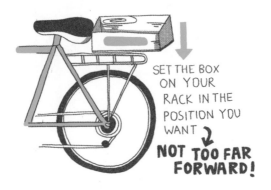

SET THE BOX ON YOUR RACK IN THE POSITION YOU WANT

NOT TOO FAR FORWARD!

1. Flip your crate over and position the mending plates on the bottom of the crate where you will want them positioned when you bolt the crate down.

2. Using the mending plate as a guide, drill through the outer hole on the right of the mending plate all the way through the bottom of the box. Before drilling the outer hole on the left, put a bolt through the first hole to keep the plate in place while drilling the second hole. Once you have drilled the second hole, remove the bolt and nut from the first hole.

3. Repeat the process with the second mending plate.

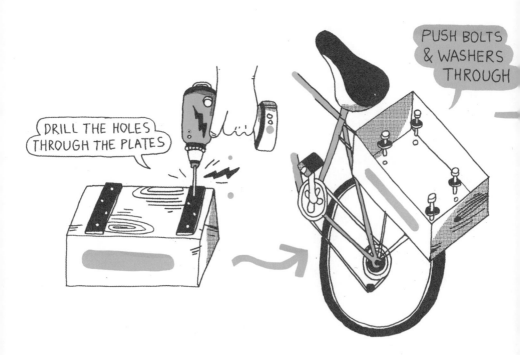

4. If your crate has a solid base (as opposed to slats), drill a few additional holes evenly distributed around the crate. This will allow water to drain out when it rains.

5. Flip your crate back over and place it on your rack. Position the mending plates underneath the bike rack, so that the rack is between the mending plate and the crate.

6. Using a screwdriver or drill fitted with a screwdriver bit, screw in the bolts, slide on the washers, and then screw the nuts underneath the mending plate. Use the wrench to gently tighten the nuts so that the crate is securely in place.

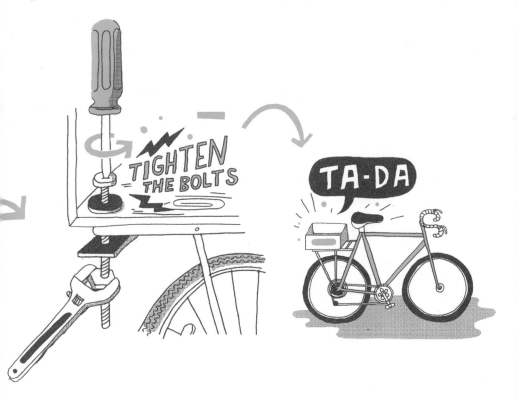

HOW SHOULD I RIDE?

If there's one thing to remember about riding a bicycle, it's this: safety first and, after that, respect. Be sure to set a good example. See that cyclist with her headphones on, blowing through the stop sign without looking left or right? No, thank you. Inconsiderate cyclists give all the other cyclists a bad name, and in a world where we want to see more people on bicycles, we need cyclists to have a good name. That means we need more well-behaved cyclists.

This doesn't mean that you won't find yourself breaking the rules sometimes—the safest route isn't always the legal one—but it does mean that you want to respect not only the rules of the road—the letter of the law—but also the other cyclists, drivers, and pedestrians around you. Remember that, ultimately, safety is subjective; there's no guide-book to tell you which situations are safer than others. A good rider is one who learns to read the road and respond accordingly. And one who makes himself or herself visible. Never assume that cars, or other cyclists, or pedestrians know your next move. Always be clear about signaling where you want to go, and try your best not to make quick, sudden movements. Unless, of course, you're avoiding a car that wasn't paying attention and is about to run you over.

A good rule of thumb is to think of yourself as a car, and follow the rules of the road just as the other drivers should. That means signaling, with plenty of lead time, when you want to turn, and stopping at stop signs. There are situations in which cyclists will argue that yielding rather than stopping is their best bet safety-wise; whatever you decide, remember that it's just as easy to get a ticket on a bicycle as in a car. Police officers aren't usually open to the "it felt safer to break the law" reasoning. If you want to know exactly which laws apply to you as a cyclist, visit bikeleague.org/StateBikeLaws, where the League of American Cyclists maintains an extensive state-by-state list.

When it comes to riding on sidewalks, this depends on where you live. In some cities, cycling on the sidewalk is illegal; others allow you to pedal as long as you are going the same speed as a pedestrian. For the record, it's actually quite hard to do this and stay upright. As always, think about your own safety and those of pedestrians. Are you really safer up on the sidewalk, or are you creating a nuisance? Sometimes street traffic is so hectic that you have to get off and walk your bike along a sidewalk; if this keeps you alive and out of danger, then it's a good choice, but be respectful of who you are sharing the sidewalk with, and don't just create more danger.

In general, riding with traffic is a good move, though there are cities where bike lanes are set up on one-way streets in the opposite direction of the movement of traffic. Remember that you are not as visible as an automobile. Just as you *always* use bike lights to be seen at night, make sure that, any time you ride, you do everything you can to make yourself visible. This means being aware of blind spots, particularly with larger vehicles like trucks. These can be deadly to cyclists, so it's important to avoid them. Always be careful when you are just behind a vehicle, or passing it, and when you are stopped at a sign or light, be sure to put yourself in front of the vehicle to be sure that you are in sight.

A smart cyclist pays attention to traffic and also to parked cars. If you ride too close to parked cars, you can easily get "doored"—the term for what happens when a driver opens the door just as you pass, either hitting you with the door, or forcing you to ride straight into the door. Sometimes, particularly if a bike lane is right next to a section of parked cars, you don't have the option of putting more distance in between you and them. In this case, *slow down* and try to be extra alert.

Using and understanding bike lanes

A bike lane is a godsend. But not all bike lanes are created equal.

The main difference between bike lanes is whether they are protected or not. A protected bike lane has a physical barrier separating cyclists and moving traffic. Conventional bike lanes in North America, however, are often not much more than a painted strip on the ground.

Here are a few of the distinctions for the various types of bike lanes:

PROTECTED BIKE LANES

These are the bike lanes you'll really love to ride in. The ones that are completely separated from the street, with some kind of physical barrier. They're usually what people are talking about when they say "If only I lived in [insert European bike capital here] I would ride all the time; the bike lanes are amazing." Why are they amazing? Because they're like bike highways, made for bicycles and bicycles only. Certainly, you still have to be a smart and safe rider, but getting in a fender bender with a fellow cyclist is entirely different from having a truck run into you.

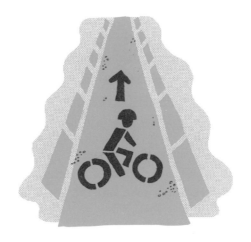

ONE-WAY AND TWO-WAY PROTECTED BIKE LANES

These are two distinct kinds of protected bike lanes. In a one-way protected bike lane, everyone is riding in the same direction. In a two-lane protected bike lane, riders are riding in both directions, kind of like a two-way mini "bicycle street." Because two-way bike lanes take up more space, they are more common on wider streets.

CONVENTIONAL BIKE LANE

This is what most people think of when they think of a bike lane in North America: a narrow section of the road designated for cyclists and identified by paint. In other words, a bike lane painted on the pavement. What separates you from the motor vehicles is a strip of paint—which, while a step in the right direction, isn't the preferred type of bike lane for most cyclists, for the obvious safety reasons, as there is nothing physically stopping a driver from entering the bike lane.

BUFFERED BIKE LANE

The idea of buffered bike lanes—putting a barrier between vehicles and cyclists—is the same as protected bike lanes, but the practice is a little different. Here, the barrier isn't physical, it's painted, like a conventional bike lane, except with additional space allotted for the buffer to give cyclists just a little more room between themselves and the vehicles in traffic.

BIKE ROUTES

Some cities will identify certain streets as part of a bike route. There may not be an actual lane painted, but they are identified as streets with less traffic, and hence safer for cyclists. They may be marked by a bicycle painted on the ground. Often you can find city-specific maps that will show these routes.

LEARN TO READ THE ROADS AND BIKE LANES

Regardless of whether you're in a protected bike lane or just on a normal street, reading the road will make you a good cyclist. Obstacles that might have little effect on you in a car can have a huge effect on you when you are on your bike. We're talking potholes, branches, trash, and so on. While you are riding, you must keep an eye on what's ahead of you so you can avoid rough patches in the road and loose objects.

The etiquette of cycling

While a fellow cyclist isn't going to pull you over for breaking a bike law, there are some general unwritten rules that considerate cyclists follow; knowing them will help you to be a better part of the flow of both bike and general automobile traffic.

TURNING AND SIGNALING

Just as when you're driving a car, when you're cycling you should signal well in advance when you intend to make a turn. Be aware of the traffic around you, and don't make any abrupt movements without first looking to see if there's a risk of getting hit. Keep an eye on who is in front of you, behind you, and to your sides, and remember that cars are usually going much faster than you are.

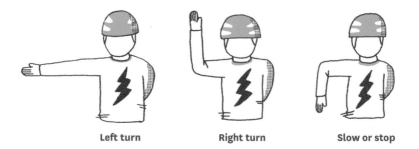

Left turn   **Right turn**   **Slow or stop**

For a left turn, extend your left arm straight out and perpendicular to your body. For a right turn, extend your left arm out, bend your elbow 90-degrees, and point your hand vertically to the sky. This is done because your left side is most often where the cars are. That being said, there is debate within the cycling community as to whether this turn signal is counterintuitive to drivers; you can also extend your right arm out so that it's perpendicular to your body, as you would with your left arm to signal a left-hand turn. To indicate slowing down or stopping, extend your left arm out and bend your elbow 90-degrees, pointing your hand to the ground.

PASSING OTHER CYCLISTS

On a long and lonely country road, passing isn't really an issue, but when you're navigating urban streets, it's an entirely different matter. Inevitably, you will come to a point where you want—sometimes even need—to pass another cyclist. Pass only if you have enough room to do so safely. That means having enough room on either the left or ride side of the cyclist in front of you so that you can pass safely. And, of course, consider what's happening on the road up ahead. In general, try to pass on the left, just as you would in a car.

The beauty of cycling as opposed to driving a car is that you can have actual exchanges with your fellow riders on the road. So when you plan to pass, a friendly "on your left" or "on your right" will alert the person you are overtaking that they have someone passing by them. Be aware, though, that when a person turns their head to look behind them, their bike goes in that direction. If a cyclist hears "on your left" and chooses to look back to see what exactly is coming up on their left, they may swerve into your path, so you want to be sure to allow ample passing room. Consider yourself warned.

Some people find bell ringing by cyclists obnoxious. Others find it necessary to alert people that there's a bicycle coming. Ringing a bell is a way of alerting other cyclists and pedestrians of your presence. How cyclists alert others to their presence can differ. I've even seen cyclists ride with a whistle in their mouth, ready to blow as hard as they can whenever anything gets in the way. Again, this is a question of both safety and respect. You want to warn people that there is a cyclist in the vicinity, but there is a difference between a *Hi! There's a cyclist behind you!* ting-ting of the bell and a *Get the hell out of my way or I'm gonna run you over* jangling. Try to be respectful and polite when you have time and space.

PREPARE FOR THE WORST

A good cyclist is a proactive cyclist, one who pays attention to traffic, respects his or her fellow cyclists, pedestrians, and, yes, drivers, and takes care of his or her bicycle to make sure it performs at its very best. But even the best of cyclists get into accidents.

When you ride a bicycle, you should be doing everything in your power to not get into an accident. Why do you constantly watch out for cars? You don't want to get run over. That's also why you choose a quiet street over a busy one. Every decision in the mind of a cyclist is made to minimize risk.

But accidents do happen, and it's best to accept that someday you may be in one. Knowing what could potentially happen will help you be prepared for such an incident.

What to do if you are in an accident

The severity of accidents varies, of course. You can fall on a set of railroad tracks because you didn't cross them at the right angle. (Trust me, I've been there.) You can run over a twig that then gets caught in your wheel, spilling you onto the pavement. You can have something come loose on your bicycle while riding. You can get "doored," that awful encounter that happens when you are calmly cycling along and someone in a parked car opens their door without looking to see if someone is coming.

An accident can happen at any time, and while many are preventable, others are not. I hope you will never be in the kind of accident where you are not physically able to respond to the situation, but if you are, hope that you've earned enough bike karma that someone will come to your assistance.

To better handle a bike-car accident in which you aren't too injured to react to the situation, here are some key things to remember.

PLAN AHEAD

Accidents are, by definition, unplanned, but just as you can better deal with bike theft (also unplanned) by being prepared for the possibility, you can do the same for accidents. When you're riding, always carry a form of identification, as well as an insurance card or policy number and emergency contact information so first responders know who to call if necessary.

YOUR FIRST RESPONSE

If you're able to move, make sure that you can get to a safe place; don't stay in the middle of the road. However, make a mental note of where you were and where your bike was at the time of the accident. If you can, take a picture of the bike before moving it. You want to get as much evidence from the scene as possible to be able to document what happened.

Just as you would after a car accident, if medical assistance arrives, don't refuse it. Allow yourself to be checked out by a medical professional on the scene.

GET AS MUCH INFORMATION AS POSSIBLE

Though you may be shaken up after an accident, you want to be sure to get as much information as possible. Here are the essentials:

→ Make, model, color, and license number of the vehicle. Do this first; if the driver ends up driving away, this will be your only evidence. This is where a cell phone becomes essential; use it to take photos of the vehicle.

→ The driver's license number and insurance information. If you are injured, ask someone to help you do this.

→ The names and information of any witnesses. If you are injured, ask someone to help you do this.

CHECK YOUR BICYCLE

If you are physically unharmed and still able to ride, that doesn't necessarily mean that you should just continue on your way. First make sure that your bicycle is safe to ride. Inspect the frame to see if you can identify anything that's broken, bent, or cracked. Give each wheel a spin and check that the brakes work. You don't want to leave the scene of one accident only to get in another one. And remember that after an accident, while you may not be physically harmed, you may be quite emotionally shaken up, and this can affect how you ride. Do not feel bad about finding another way to get home, perhaps by calling a friend or a cab to come and get you.

DOCUMENT ALL THE INFORMATION YOU HAVE

After you get home, while the accident is still fresh in your mind, write down everything you can remember. This way you will have your best recollection of the accident on hand in the event that you need it later. Put this together with all the driver and witness contact information.

If you have to get medical attention, keep a record of all of the information, as well as any receipts for treatment.

CONSULT AN ATTORNEY

Bike and car accidents are complex. Don't try to take on the insurance companies by yourself. It's always best to get the help of a professional.

What Would a Lawyer Do?

Daniel Flanzig is a personal injury lawyer in New York City who specializes in bike-related cases. He and his counterparts at New York Bike Lawyer also developed a bike crash app for smartphones, which, in the event of an accident, helps you to collect all of the critical data that a lawyer will need to help you. Here are his tips for what to do when you get in an accident.

1. Call the police and insist that a report is made. This will ensure that you have the proper identity of the driver and vehicle owner. If you don't call the police, make sure you have the license plate number of the vehicle.

2. Use a GoPro or other recording device, like your smartphone. A video to record the scene before and after it happens—if you are willing to record every time you ride— is the best evidence you can ask for.

3. Don't repair or discard your bike or other key evidence. It may be needed if you file a claim.

4. Have you checked your own auto policy? Verify whether you have sufficient uninsured or underinsured motorist coverage, also known as SUM coverage. This will help you if the driver involved in the accident is not properly insured.

5. Don't give a statement to an insurance company until you speak to an attorney. Most attorneys give free consultations, so there is no cost for calling and getting some free advice.

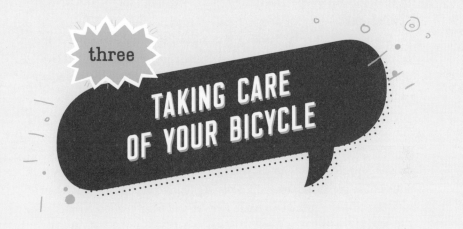

three

TAKING CARE OF YOUR BICYCLE

A bicycle—be it a rusty old Schwinn that dates back to before you were born or a multi-thousand-dollar road bike that's sure to make you win races—is a machine that needs love. Take care of it, and it will take care of you. Let it sit on the porch through the entire rainy season, without so much as a spin around the block, and it may not be so nice to you.

While different bicycles may require different levels of care—your around-town bicycle may need a little less love than a finely tuned mountain bike—one thing is sure: you can't forget about your bicycle's needs.

But where to begin? Parking it in a good spot and keeping it out of the rain—that's easy enough to accomplish, but what about all those other things? There are two words that tend to intimidate many new cyclists, and even the seasoned two-wheeled crowd:

bike maintenance.

It's time we all got a little more comfortable with bike maintenance, not just for the sake of our bicycles, but for our own sake, too. Few skills in life are as empowering as being able to change a flat on your own. When you know a few basic tweaks and fixes you can master with your bicycle, with just a handful of essential tools and a little elbow grease, you're unstoppable.

But before we get there, let's talk about bike shops. Ever gotten a flat and felt silly for walking into a bike shop because you didn't have the right tools with you to change it yourself? That's okay; every cyclist has been there. If you don't know how to change a flat, don't beat yourself up. That doesn't make you any less of a cyclist. Keep reading and learn how to fix that flat, because there's nothing quite like being on a ride, hearing a tire go "pop," and knowing that you can take care of the problem all on your own.

But rest assured, you don't have to learn how to do it all—and when you don't know how to do a maintenance or repair item yourself, bike shops are there to help.

HOW DO I FIND A GOOD BIKE SHOP?

What should you look for in a good bike shop? Here are a few things to consider.

Proximity

Most people choose a bike shop simply because it's close by, and that makes perfect sense. Especially if you live in a city, where you probably have a choice of bike shops, keep it local. There's no point in driving across town with your trusty two-wheeled steed if you can get the work done next door. That being said, there *are* some factors that might lure you across town.

A good fit for you

A good bike shop is the one that makes you feel comfortable, the one that you want to go into. It's the one that makes you feel at home, no matter what your cycling level. To find out whether your local shop is *that* shop, have a conversation; ask questions.

The golden rule

Bike mechanics are there to help you, but that doesn't mean you get to be a jerk. If you want good service, you have to be a respectful customer. That means coming in when you say you're going to come in, and knowing what you're coming in for. Bike mechanics have busy schedules, and if you call ahead to get a chain repaired but then saunter in and ask to have your tires changed and your brakes checked as well, you are going to end up with a cranky mechanic. If you add work to their list, it affects the next person on the repair schedule. In other words, when you call to schedule a time to get your bike worked on, tell them everything you can about what's wrong with your bicycle or what you need done so that they can determine how much time to allocate for the work. Happy mechanic, happy bicycle, happy rider; it all comes full circle. And while it's not customary, bike mechanics also do appreciate tips, even if they come in the form of homemade cookies or a six-pack of craft beer.

But what if your bicycle is just making a funny sound and you actually don't know what work you need done? A lot of bike shops offer free estimates, which allows you to bring your bicycle in for an assessment so that you know what you are getting into before you go in for the official service.

COMMUNITY BIKE SHOPS

Some cities have not only bike stores but also community bike shops or bike cooperatives. Their exact functions may vary, but in general they are set up as social enterprises, intended to build community and be a resource for anyone with a love of cycling. Often these places are set up so that you can bring in your bike not just to get it worked on but so you can work on it yourself. There may be volunteers who can help you figure out what your bike needs and how to do it, and an array of bike tools and workspace so that you can work more comfortably on your bicycle than, let's say, in your kitchen. These are great places for people who want to feel empowered to work on their bicycles themselves but don't have the space or all the tools at home. Often community bike shops offer workshops and classes, the perfect place to master your bike

Bike Shop Vocabulary

Need the right language to navigate the bike shop? Here are a few essential terms that a bike mechanic might use when talking about your bicycle.

CASSETTE → The cluster of sprockets that's on your back wheel.

CHAINRING → The sprockets of the crankset, of which there may be one, two, or three.

CRANKSET → The part of the bicycle that takes your pedaling power and uses that power to drive the back wheel. It's what your pedals are attached to.

DERAILLEUR → The mechanism that allows you to change gears.

FORK → The part that holds the front wheel.

FRAME → The main structure of your bicycle; essentially what is left if everything else—wheels, handlebars, seat, and so on—is stripped off.

HEADSET → The part at the front of the bicycle where the handlebar stem and fork are fitted.

PINCH FLAT → A flat you get from the bike tube's being pinched between the tire and the rim. Also called a "snake-bite flat."

PRESTA → A valve that is smaller in diameter than the Schrader, common on road bikes. Presta tubes can be used in holes drilled for Schrader valves, but not vice versa.

PSI → Stands for "pounds per square inch," the unit of measure for tire inflation. Often marked on your bike tire, next to the size.

SCHRADER → The type of valve on a bike tire tube. It's the same valve as those used on automobile tires.

STEM → The part that connects the handlebars to the bicycle.

maintenance skills, and there is an emphasis on repurposing materials, so you will probably find used bike parts as opposed to new ones. These can provide some added flair and personality to your bicycle.

If you are interested in the concept of community bike shops and want to find out if there is one close to you, an excellent online resource is bikecollectives.org. They even have information for people interested in launching their own community bike shop. So if there isn't one close to you, why not launch your own? If you build it, the cyclists will come.

···

GENERAL BICYCLE CARE YOU CAN EASILY DO
···

Your bicycle doesn't need all the bells and whistles of fine-tuned bike maintenance every single day of its life. But it does need some regular care. Just as we humans try to eat well, get enough exercise and sleep, and find a nice balance between work and play so that we stay healthy and happy, so too our bicycles need some regular care and maintenance.

Your regular bike maintenance should include the following:

Keep it clean

Bikes get dirty; having a bike with some dirt on it does show it's used and loved, and there's no need to keep it sparkling and pristine. But it's good to wash it every once in a while. Spent the afternoon on an especially muddy trail? Give your bicycle a rinse off when you get home, being sure to use the most gentle hose pressure possible, as you don't want to force water where it can do damage. Even if you ride mostly on urban streets, giving your bike a good wipe-down once in a while is a good habit to get into, because keeping your bicycle clean—especially the chain and sprockets, which are subject to the most wear on a bicycle—ensures that it runs smoothly and has a longer life.

Lube the chain

Buy some bicycle chain lube (you want lube that is specifically made for this purpose, as other types of oil can make your chain quite filthy) at a local bike shop, find a clean rag, and give your chain a good lube. How often you need to lube your chain depends on how much you use your bicycle. If the chain is particularly grimy, it may also need a good wash with warm water and dish soap. See page 70 for more detailed instructions.

Check your brakes

It's terrifying to be riding fast down a hill and realize you are going to have to drag your feet on the ground to come to a full stop. But even if your brakes are working, they may not be functioning as well as they could. Make a monthly habit of checking the brakes; that way you can be pretty sure your brakes will never fail you. To check your brake levers, simply pull them toward the handlebars. When the brake levers are squeezed, there should be an inch or more between the levers and the handlebars. If you squeeze them and have to pull them closer to the handlebars to fully engage the brakes, the brakes need to be tightened. To make your bike mechanic happy (see "Extra things your bike mechanic really wishes you would do," page 63), check your brake pads too. Riding in a climate where it rains a lot? Note that rainy riding makes your brakes wear out much faster, so you'll have to be more vigilant.

Check your lights

If you're already in the habit of always keeping your bike lights with you (because you never know when you'll be cycling in the dark), then also get into the habit of checking the light batteries. Try to check them on a monthly basis. If the light is starting to flicker or it's not as bright as it used to be, switch out the batteries for new ones. Often that's all you need to do, but if your lights are old, it may be the bulb, and it just might be time for a new light.

Check your tires

Checking your tires for wear and tear at home can prevent you from having to deal with a flat while out on a ride. A tire that is so worn that the tread is completely worn down is a flat tire waiting to happen. Time to take that tire in for an upgrade.

Get a yearly checkup

Unless you are a trained bike mechanic, be sure to take that bicycle of yours to a professional once a year. Drop it off, tell the bike shop the bicycle needs its annual checkup, and when you pick it up, it will be running like new. If you've ridden your bicycle hard, or if you haven't been good about caring for it, a few parts and pieces may need to get switched out—something to keep in mind when you are budgeting for the checkup fee. Also keep in mind that all modern drivetrains require the chain to be replaced every 1,200 to 1,500 miles; if this doesn't happen, you're going to damage the cassette and chainrings pretty quickly, which will lead to a much pricier replacement. Think of it this way: an annual visit to the bike mechanic ensures your bicycle a long and happy life.

EXTRA THINGS YOUR BIKE MECHANIC REALLY WISHES YOU WOULD DO

It's easy to take your bike into a shop to get it worked on, but bike mechanics are people, too, and they prefer working on bikes that get some love at home. Tori Bortman knows all about at-home and in-the-shop mechanics. As the owner of Gracie's Wrench, she empowers people to get to know their bikes and do some of their own work on them. Working as a bike mechanic, Bortman has a list of things that she, and every other bike mechanic out there, wishes you would do. It's great advice not only for making sure that you take care of your bicycle, but also to ensure that you build a solid relationship with your mechanic and keep them happy working on your two wheels.

Pay attention to your rims

In rainy, wet, or humid weather, metal rims get coated with a horrible black grime. When you have your bike upside down to oil the chain, use a clean, dry towel to wipe the grime away. This simple act can add another year or more to the life of your wheels (which are the most expensive part of your bike).

Pay attention to your brake pads

When your brakes aren't working, often it's because your pads are worn down. Pads have wear indicators—little divots in the pad that you can easily see. If they are barely visible—or worse, you can't see them at all—it's time to get the brake pads replaced. If your pads seem worn, make an appointment with the shop before they ruin your rim or destroy your brake cables by pulling too hard on your brakes, trying to make them work.

Clean up your bike before you bring it in

Your bike runs better when it's clean, and it's also easier to fix when it's clean. Do you shower before a doctor's appointment or a massage? Treat your mechanic and your bike with the same respect. A simple shower with a very light pressure hose and some soapy water will help get it clean before you bring it to the shop.

Schedule regular appointments if you're riding a lot

Put a reminder on your calendar to make an appointment every six months to a year if you're riding over two thousand miles annually. (To figure this out, multiply the average number of times you ride each week, times your average miles in a ride, times fifty-two.) If these are commuter miles, which are a lot rougher on your bike, schedule service every six months. This way you don't let parts wear too far and need replacement.

No offense!

Don't be offended when a mechanic tells you everything that's wrong with your bike. It's not that they're trying to gouge you; rather, they're trying to save you from having to come back three times in one month for different problems. You can always refuse a service that's not necessary, but the mechanic is just letting you know what to expect and giving you the chance to do some preventive maintenance.

Don't wait until a strange noise gets really bad

If you notice something strange or out of the norm with your bike, don't assume that it's just you or that it will go away on its own. This is how little problems get to be big, expensive problems. If you think something is wrong, swing by the shop and have them take a look. Estimates are usually free and can save you money down the road.

. . . .
DIY BIKE MAINTENANCE
. . . .

We're still working on those two important words: *bike maintenance.* But now we're talking about what you can learn to do on your own in the way of tune-ups, repairs, and replacements. There are a few of these things that don't require a degree in rocket science. One great benefit is that doing a few things at home regularly makes life a lot easier for your bike mechanic when you do have to take your bicycle in for a bigger overhaul.

You don't need official bike mechanic training to learn how to do bike maintenance at home. For visual learners, the Internet is full of helpful videos for all sorts of problems you may encounter with your bicycle. If you want to be more empowered to work on your bicycle, consider taking a bike maintenance class. These are an excellent way to master the necessary skills with the help of a professional. Ask your local bike shop or bike club if they organize this kind of thing. Lessons are a terrific introduction—after that, the best way to master these things is to practice, practice, practice. And remember, the bicycle is, at its core, a simple and sturdy machine. Be gentle, don't push on things too hard, but don't be afraid that loosening a screw is going to make the entire thing fall apart.

And if you get in over your head? Take the bike to a bike shop. Whatever your bike problem is, there's always an answer, and when things get too complicated, there is no shame in asking a professional.

Bike maintenance tools to have at home

If you don't already have them, investing in a few tools and supplies will help make home maintenance much easier. The following are what you will want to have on hand for any kind of work on your bike, be it adjusting a seat that doesn't have a quick release or changing a flat.

PATCH KIT

Just because you've gotten a hole in your bike tube doesn't mean that you need to throw it away. A patch kit lets you repair a flat tire while on the road.

HEX WRENCH SET

Also referred to as an Allen wrench or hex key, this is an essential tool for the bicycle, as it's used for everything from adjusting the seat post to tightening the brakes. While "loose" hex keys allow for more flexibility and enable you to handle a wider range of home-based bike maintenance tasks, for quick fixes on a bike, a hex wrench set or multitool that has a few sizes in one tool can work wonders. It's also easily transportable.

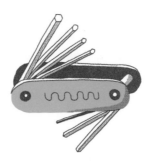

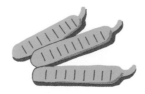

TIRE LEVERS

These simple tools are made to ease the process of removing the tire from the rim and putting it back on when you get a flat and need to replace the tube. They generally come in a set of three.

FLOOR PUMP

You'll want this when pumping up that new and improved tire. It's called a floor pump because it stands on the floor, as opposed to smaller pumps that are made for taking along on rides. Those are great for fixing a flat on the road, but investing in a heavy-duty floor pump for use at home will make life much easier. If you're planning on doing a lot of long bicycle rides, get a mini pump that you can take along to fix a flat while on the road.

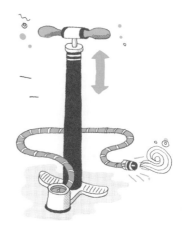

OLD TOOTHBRUSH

You'd be surprised how handy this is for cleaning the chain and sprockets and even for getting rid of the mud that's caked into all the nooks and crannies. (Be sure to stash your bike brush absolutely nowhere near your actual toothbrush!)

CHAIN LUBE

I mentioned this earlier in "Lube the chain." Keeping the chain lubed is one of the easiest and most helpful things that you can do to keep your bike happy and healthy. Again, be sure to buy lube that is specifically made for this purpose.

OLD RAGS

Don't discard those old T-shirts—ripped up into rags, they are helpful for applying lube, washing the chain, and a variety of other bike maintenance tasks. It's nice to have something to wipe your hands on, and trust me, you don't want to be wiping them on your jeans.

HAND CLEANER

Speaking of wiping your hands, the lingering residue of bike grease isn't the same as good old garden dirt, and you may find that the cleanup is a bit more difficult. To quickly clean those greasy hands, start with regular dish soap, which will work well if you've got a little chain lube on your hands. You're greasier than that? Then invest in some cleaner that cuts grease. There are bicycle-specific ones available, but you can use the same hand cleaners you find in automotive stores.

Bike maintenance you can learn to do on your own

While no one is going to require you to know how to do these things at home, they are fairly easy tasks to learn and master. Put them into practice, and when you take your bicycle in for its yearly checkup you will make your bike mechanic very happy.

HOW TO CHANGE THE HANDLEBAR TAPE

If you have a road bike, old handlebar tape can get grimy or even start flaking off. That's not so enjoyable to grip on a ride, so for an easy uplift to your cycling experience, remove the old handlebar tape and put on new stuff.

Handlebar tape comes in a variety of colors, and you can even get tape made from cork, which can give your bicycle a nice natural, vintage look. Start at the end of the handlebar, leaving a little extra tape, about half the width, hanging over the end. This will be stuffed into the end with a bar plug when you are finished. Wrap upward and outward (winding clockwise on the right side and counter clockwise on the left). Take off the adhesive backing little by little as you go, or you'll end up in a sticky situation (pun intended). Wrap tightly, with each full circle covering a third to half of the tape that's already on the handlebar. If it's not tight, or there are gaps, pull the tape away and do it again. When you get to the brake lever, pull up the hoods, and wrap the tape in a figure eight around it (this won't be visible when you pull the hood back). When you wrap the top of the handlebar, be sure to wrap toward the bicycle seat. When you get to the top of the handlebars, use electrical tape to tape down the end of the handlebar tape.

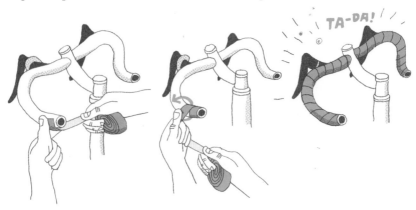

HOW TO CLEAN AND GREASE THE SEAT POST

If you have never cleaned or greased the seat post, chances are it may just be stuck. But it doesn't have to be that way. It's good, every once in a while, to remove the seat and clean inside the tube. Important: before you do this, be sure to mark your seat post height so that you can easily put it back exactly where it was. You can use electrical tape or even etch a mark into the seat post. Now loosen it up, take the seat out, and use a rag to clean out the inside of the seat tube. Add some grease, replace the seat, and you're good to go.

HOW TO LUBE THE CHAIN

A clean and lubed chain is a happy chain, and you'll also notice that pedaling is much smoother. To clean the chain, a chain cleaner can come in handy, but isn't necessary. If you're good about cleaning the chain and there are just a few spots that are a bit gunky, you can scrub that out from individual chain links with just your designated old toothbrush, or if need be, a little soap and water. Once the chain is clean, it needs lube.

Apply a little bit of lube every few chain links, then spin the pedal so that the chain goes all the way around, and the lube is now lubricating the entire chain and cassette. Wipe the excess chain lubricant off with a rag; less oil is much better than too much oil. Now that the chain is clean and lubed, keep it that way. Wipe the chain off regularly with a rag; this helps it stay clean and prevents a buildup of too much gunk everywhere.

The first bike fix that any two-wheeled lifer should learn is how to change a flat. You'll want to master this either in the comfort of your own home or at a community bike shop where you have someone helping you. Because the side of the road is a much less comfortable spot to learn in.

Flats are far less common with newer, higher-quality tires. These are expensive, of course, but they mean that you can nearly eliminate flats. This is good news for anyone who doesn't want to deal with flats or has a bicycle whose tires are a real pain to change, like a bicycle with an internally geared hub (with gears inside rather than outside the hub).

Changing a flat is simple in theory but can be hard in practice if you're not used to doing it. The basics are removing the wheel, then the tube, patching or replacing it, putting it back in, putting the tire back on, and pumping it up. This can become difficult when you're removing the tire from the rim and later when getting everything back into place, but with a little practice this too can become an easy routine. Here's how it's done on the front wheel (specifics for the rear wheel follow). Also, be sure to check out the illustrations on pages 74–75.

1. Release the brakes, then release the wheel from the fork—the wheel is held to the fork by the wheel axle. You will have either a quick-release system or a bolt-on axle, which needs to be removed with a wrench. This is much easier to do if you turn the bike upside down so that the handlebars and seat are on the ground.

2. The tire is held in place inside the rim by pressure; the section where the tire meets the rim is called the tire bead. To remove

the tire and gain access to the bike tube, you need to relieve that pressure. Start by getting any remaining air out of the tire by depressing the valve.

3. To loosen the tire bead from the rim, push the side of the tire wall in toward the center of the rim, or pinch the tire on both sides. Doing this, work your way around the whole tire.

4. When there is enough slack in the tire, pop the edge of the tire over the rim. This is where tire levers can come in very handy (as mentioned earlier, tire levers generally come in packs of three, because that is the most you will need to change a tire). If you're using levers, start opposite the tire valve (which you want to avoid damaging) and use the tire lever to pry the tire bead up and over the edge of the rim. Hook the tire lever to the spoke, then insert an additional lever about two or three spokes down from the first one. You want the tire to be loose enough that you can run a tire lever around the entire rim, pulling one side of the tire over it, and leaving the other side in the rim. If necessary, place a third lever, spaced an additional two or three spokes away from the middle one; this will cause the middle one to come out. Keep repeating this until the tire is loose enough.

5. When the tire bead is free from the rim, you should be able to loosen the rest by hand. You do not need to take the entire tire off; while you pull one side of the tire up and over the rim, leave the other side of the tire in.

6. Remove the tube by first removing the valve from the rim, then pulling the rest of the tube out. Determine where the tube is punctured, and when you find the spot, locate the same area on

the tire, to make sure that whatever made the puncture isn't still in the tire. Then run your fingers (carefully) around the inside of the tire to make sure there are no foreign objects stuck inside that would cause more punctures once you have put the tube back in.

7. When you are ready to put the repaired tube or a new tube back in, partially inflate the tube to give it some shape.

8. Make sure one side of the tire is in place against the rim. Starting with the valve stem, place the tube inside the tire.

9. Once the tube is in, make sure the valve is straight; this is important, as you don't want a bent valve. Starting close to the valve, put the tire back in place, so that the tire bead is positioned inside the rim. This will get harder (much harder) as you make your way around the tire.

10. Pinch both sides of the tire to get the final section of tire in place inside the rim, or use bike levers for help. Make sure that the bike tube isn't pinched anywhere between the tire and the rim, as this could lead to yet another flat.

11. Inflate the tire partially and check that it is not pinched between the bead and rim by pinching in on both sides of the tire all the way around the circumference. Then fully inflate the tire—and get back to riding!

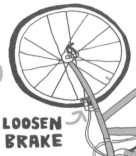

FLIP TO START

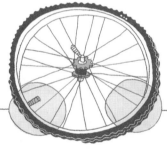

REMOVE WHEEL

LOOSEN BRAKE

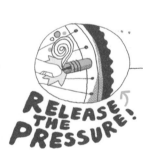

RELEASE THE PRESSURE!

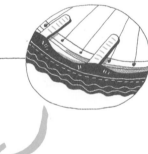

REMOVE THE TUBE

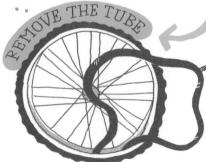

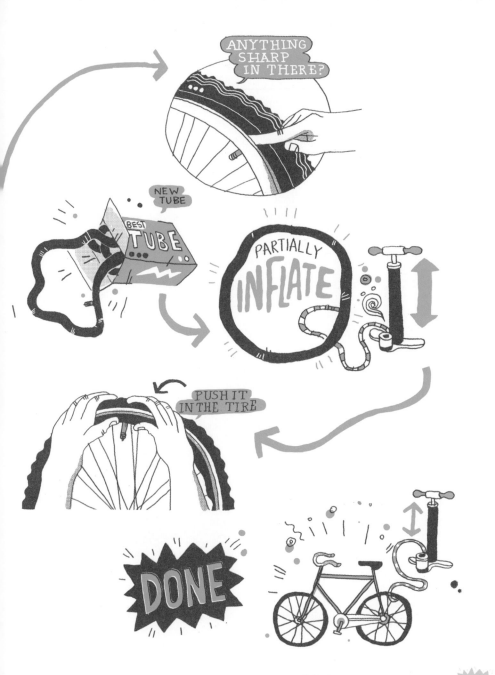

The process for changing the rear wheel is the same, except that if you are riding a bicycle with gears you will need to do a couple of additional things. As with changing the front tire, if you don't have a bicycle repair stand, this can be easier if you turn the bicycle upside down. Shift so that the chain is down to the smallest cog, then turn your bicycle upside down. Release the brake and the quick release on the axle and push the wheel out. If it doesn't easily come out of the derailleur, you can pull the derailleur back with your finger. Once you have repaired or replaced the tube, put the wheel back on. Push down on the derailleur and put the chain on the smallest ring. Pull the wheel into the frame and make sure it's straight, then secure the quick release.

WHAT TO DO IF YOU GET A FLAT ON A RIDE

If you get a flat while out on a bicycle ride, stop and assess the situation. Examine the tire, looking for any signs of a puncture or the object that caused the flat, because if a sharp object has pierced the tire to puncture the tube, chances are it's still there, and you want to remove it before putting in a patched or new tube.

Can't see the culprit? It's time to remove the wheel from the bicycle and take the tire off so that you can replace the tube. Once you have gotten the tire off, carefully look on the inside of the tire walls for glass, a nail, or anything else that may be the culprit. Often it's something small, like a thorn, that may have penetrated the tire and punctured the tube without leaving a noticeable hole in the tire wall. In this case, remove whatever made the puncture—you don't want to keep riding with a piece of glass in your tire, do you?—and then you can just repair or swap the tube out and be off on your merry way.

Other times, the puncture or cut is noticeable; there may even be a large slash in the tire. In this case, you need to cover it up; if it stays open, the bike tube inside is going to remain vulnerable to more punctures. In a pinch—in other words, on a ride where you have no access to a bike shop—a dollar bill can actually work for this. Fold the dollar bill so that you can wriggle it into the tire, and it will stay in place, covering the hole. This will keep the tube from popping through the hole, letting you ride home, where you can properly deal with the problem.

WHAT SHOULD YOU DO WITH A PUNCTURED TUBE?

Inevitably, you will have a punctured tire and tube; it happens to every cyclist. Here are a few options for what to do with them.

Repair. If you're one to go on long rides away from civilization—I'm talking about those glorious Saturday rides in the countryside—carry a patch kit, an extra tube, and a mini bike pump. The extra tube can easily be switched out if you get a flat, and if you have the misfortune to get a second flat on the same ride, you have the patch kit for backup.

Once you're home and have some time on your hands, get to repairing that punctured tube. A tube can be repaired many times before you have to toss it. Usually, a punctured tire is caused by something like a nail or piece of glass, and that makes the puncture small and easy to fix.

To patch, choose a patch that's a little larger than the puncture. Roughen the surface around the puncture with some sandpaper or emery cloth. If you have a glueless patch, just put it on and apply pressure. If you're using glue or rubber cement, put a thin, smooth layer of it on the tube, then put on the patch and press firmly.

Reuse. Don't you dare throw those bike tubes away! Nowadays there are lots of independent businesses doing cool things with used bike tubes. Search around and see if anyone needs them. Those bike tubes can also be easily used for a variety of creations at home, like making your own earrings (page 85) or even a wallet (page 81).

HOW TO BUY NEW BIKE TUBES

It's nice to have a few bike tubes on hand at home so that you don't have to make a trip to the bike shop every time you need a new one. To buy the right ones, you need to know what size fits your bike tire and whether you have a presta or schrader valve. The size is marked on the side of the tire. These numbers can be a little confusing, especially given the fact that mountain bikes are almost always measured in inches and road bicycles in metric, but as a rule they refer first to the diameter of the tire and then the width of the tire.

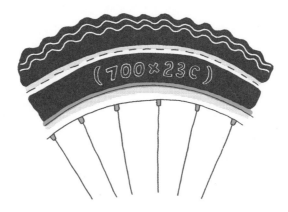

To make things even more confusing, there are two methods of measuring, so you will often see two number references printed or embossed on the tire. For example, a common road tire size is 700x23c, also written 23-622. Often bike tubes will give a range, like 700x18/23. Remember that the second number is the width of the tube, which means that this specific tube fits a tire that's between 18 and 23 millimeters in width, so it will work for any tire in that range.

Write down those numbers and take them to the bike shop. They'll be able to help you find the tubes that you need.

PUTTING BIKE PARTS TO A SECOND USE

The beauty of a bicycle is that it can be used for much more than its original purpose. A simple and fine-tuned work of engineering, a bicycle has parts that are often still usable after they have served their primary role as a part of your mode of transportation. Your bicycle continues to have a life even after its parts become old and dingy. Unlike the modern car, the design of bikes hasn't gotten much more complicated since their early days. Their simplicity means that their many components can easily be pulled apart. We're talking about bike upcycling, using parts of your beloved steed to make something new.

In the design world, as reclaimed materials become more and more popular, it's no surprise that we're seeing everyday items made from bike parts. A wheel becomes the base of a table. An old helmet is used as a planter. A bike tube lives a new life as a messenger bag.

But you don't have to be an expert designer to turn your used bike parts into new creations. Many bicycle upcycling projects are simple, and you're limited only by your imagination.

Bike Tubes

Let's start with the easiest of bike parts to upcycle: the tire tube.

First things first: if you have a punctured tube, do what you can to patch it. Always try to repair first. But when a tube is totally blown or shredded, or you're just stuck without a patch kit, don't throw those bike tubes away. If you're a fan of upcycling, bike tubes are like black gold.

If for some magical reason you or your friends aren't prone to flats, you can also ask your local bike shop for their throwaways. Much better to upcycle them into something new than have them destined for the trash.

As a material, bike tubes are very friendly. Soft and pliable, they are easy to cut, and while from afar they may look like a dark metal, they're lightweight and flexible. This makes them ideal for making a variety of things, from bracelets to bike bags. You can even cut them into long strips and knit with them. In this way, the options for bike tubes are more or less endless.

To prep bike tubes for use in any project, cut the tube lengthwise down the middle, so that you end up with one long, wide band. Wash the tube with warm water and soap and hang to dry. Once dry, the band can be rolled up and held together with a rubber band for easy storage. This also helps to keep the tubes flat, which makes measuring and cutting them a little easier.

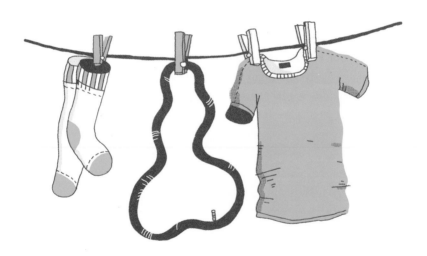

DIY Bike Tube Wallet

There are many ways you can sew a wallet, but here we stick to a simple, nonfolding design that's big enough to carry a few credit cards, your driver's license and insurance card, and some cash. For this project, wider tubes, like a mountain bike tube, work best. Bike tubes can be hard to sew in a regular sewing machine, so before you start, make sure you have the right equipment. If you don't have an industrial sewing machine, there are a few tricks that will make sewing bike tubes easier. You can use paper on either side of the bike tube to help feed it through; another easy option is to buy a Teflon, or nonstick, presser foot, which is made to sew difficult materials like suede. You also want a needle that can handle the bike tube, so opt for a sewing needle that is made for tougher, thicker fabrics like denim. The thread tension may need to be adjusted, so do a sample first before you sew your wallet. You can choose the color of thread, but note that black will match the wallet and hide sewing mistakes, while color will make for a fun detail but mistakes will be more noticeable.

TOOLS

Bike tube

Scissors

Sewing machine

Thread

1 → Cut three pieces of bike tube:
Two pieces, 2¾ inches x 3¾ inches (70 x 95 mm)
One piece, 2¾ inches x 2¾ inches (70 x 70 mm)

2 → Place one of the larger rectangles vertically so that the outside of the tube is facing outward and the short side is at the top. On the right edge of the rectangle, measure ½-inch from the top and mark with a pencil. Starting at the top left edge, cut a diagonal

CONTINUED →

line across to this point. Do the same with the small square, being sure to face the outside of the tube toward you. This cut will allow easier access to your cards and cash.

3 → Place the rectangle with the diagonal cut on top of the other rectangle piece, so that the insides of the bike tubes are touching. The bottom edges and sides should be aligned. Adjust the stitch length on your sewing machine to be longer than usual.

4 → Leaving a border of about ⅛ inch, sew the two rectangles first, sewing around three edges, leaving the side with the diagonal cut unsewn. Then add the smaller piece, with bottom edges aligned and the diagonal edges parallel. Sew a second seam close to, but not on top of the earlier one. If you have an industrial sewing machine, you may be able to sew all three layers together at the same time. Do not reverse to secure the thread ends; knot them instead. If you have used paper to feed the wallet through the sewing machine, wet the paper over the seams to make it easier to pull off without disturbing the stitches. Voilà!

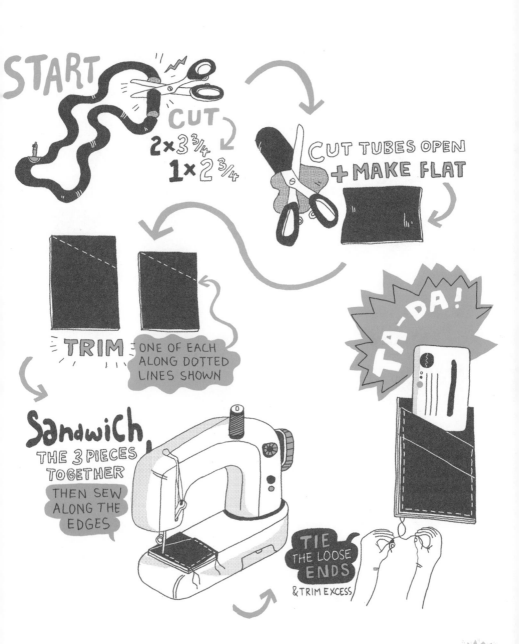

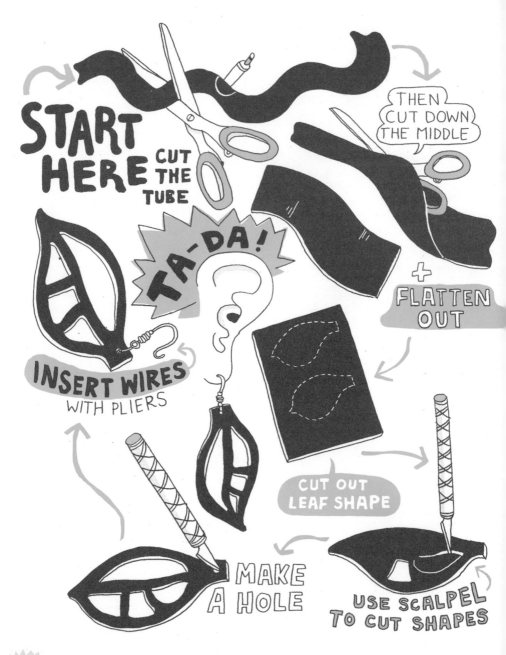

DIY Bike Tube Earrings

For anyone who likes to wear big earrings, these are lightweight no matter their size, which means your ears won't get weighed down. Note that because of the nature of the bike tube, they will curve over time.

TOOLS
Bike tube
Scissors
X-ACTO knife
Hook earring wires
Pliers

1 → Using scissors, cut the earring shape out of the tube freehand, or use a paper stencil to help guide you. Think about how long and how wide you want your earrings to be. Note that, because of the bike tube's inherent tubular shape, you will get a bit of a natural curl, so while flat, wide earrings may look good right when you cut them, they may not stay that flat for long.

2 → Cut a design with finer cuts and straight lines in the inside of the earrings with an X-ACTO knife.

3 → Once the design is cut out, use scissors or an X-ACTO knife to make a small hole at the top of the earring. With the pliers, bend the earring wire back so that you can easily insert it into the hole.

4 → Wear your earrings with pride or gift them to all of your bike-loving friends or those who need inspiration to get on two wheels.

Spokes

Did you bend or a break a spoke that has to be replaced? Don't throw the old one away! Just like bike tubes, bike spokes can be reused as well. If you have some heavy-duty pliers and a bit of arm strength, they can be bent into a variety of things, but even unbent they can be useful. Here are a few uses for both bent and unbent spokes.

USES FOR OLD SPOKES

Skewers → Thread marinated vegetables onto (clean!) old spokes (which pack easily and are great for bike trips) and pop them on the grill. Then be sure to invite all your bike friends over for a true feast.

Key chain → Bend the spoke into a funky shape (rectangle, star, and so on) and use as a key chain.

Plant markers → With a spoke and a piece of bike tube, you can label all your garden plants. Cut a rectangle out of a bike tube, then use a permanent white marker to write the plant name. Cut a small hole in the top and bottom of the rectangle, then slip the bike spoke through it and push it into the ground near the plant.

Oversized paperclips → Bend the spoke into a paperclip shape, and you can use it as a bookmark or even a money clip.

Cocktail stirrer → Give it a good cleaning first, of course.

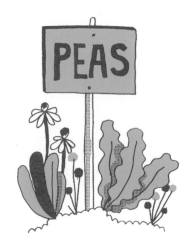

DIY Spoke Cards

Want to add a little flair to your bicycle? Make some spoke cards. Some people hate them, some people love them, but there's no denying that spoke cards do bring a little personality to a bicycle. Spoke cards can serve a variety of purposes: marking bikes taking part in a bike race, a guerilla marketing tactic, or even just simple art. Making your own is as simple as designing a card, laminating it, and wedging into your bike spokes.

TOOLS

Paper

Scissors

Laminating sheets

1 → Design your spoke card to be the size of a playing card, 2½ by 3½ inches (64 x 89 mm). The design can be a picture, a map of a bike route, an advertisement for your pedal-powered business, whatever!

2 → Print your design and cut out the card.

3 → Laminate, then cut out the card, leaving a small border of the lamination sheet around the card to protect it.

4 → Push the card in between the spokes, toward the hub so it is wedged securely in place.

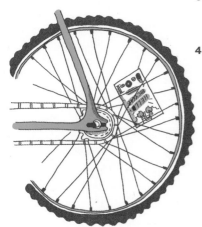

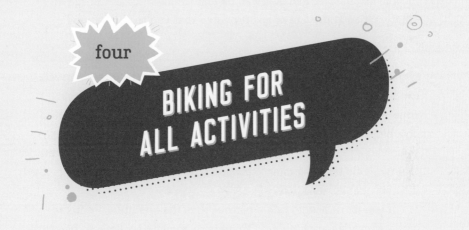

four

BIKING FOR ALL ACTIVITIES

A bicycle can serve many purposes. It can be your mode of transportation to get to work. It can be your form of exercise. It can be a way to travel. It can even be your profession. But no matter what purpose a bicycle serves in your life, one thing is for sure: cycling is fun. Whether you're on a short ride to the grocery store, on a long weekend ride with friends, or on a multi-day trip with your sleeping bag stuffed into one of your panniers, your trusty two-wheeled steed is there to carry you along, and it's going to feel great.

That feeling of uninhibited youthful exhilaration that you once felt on a bicycle is still attainable today. After all, the enjoyment of a bicycle has no age. Pedaling can be just as much fun at the age of ninety-six as at the age of six, provided that you're still in good pedaling shape.

We have lots of opportunities to trade in our four-wheeled trips for two wheels. Granted, the prospect of going some distance on a bicycle can be intimidating. But did you know that half of all the trips that Americans make by car are two miles or less? An easy average speed on a bicycle is ten to fifteen miles per hour, making that two-mile trip somewhere in the range of eight to twelve minutes. Suddenly, making that two-mile trip on a bicycle instead doesn't seem like that much of a lifestyle change, now does it?

If you know how to ride a bicycle, then the opportunities in the world of cycling are limitless. There is so much to be done, so much to be explored, and so much fun to be had. Whether you're biking to work or traveling to a new country, it can all be done by bicycle. You need only to be willing to try.

As Eddy Merckx, the famous bicycle racer, once said,

"Ride as much or as little, or as long or as short as you feel. But ride."

COMMUTING

Ever considered riding your bike to work? Then you are part of an ever-growing group of people who prefer two wheels for their commute. According to the League of American Cyclists, in the United States between 2000 and 2011 bike commuting grew by 47 percent, and overall the number of trips made by bicycle in the United States more than doubled, from 1.7 billion in 2001 to 4 billion in 2009.

As more and more cities invest in cycling infrastructure, bike commuting is a trend that can be seen in many countries around the world. As people look for ways to be more active in their everyday lives, and to do their part to decrease their impact on the environment, bike commuting is a sensible option.

How do I start bike commuting?

As that famous sporting goods company says, "Just do it." Yes, the best way to start bike commuting is simply to get on your bicycle and bike to work. As long as you have a bicycle and a job that's within a reasonable distance from home (and "reasonable distance" is up to you; some people will ride over an hour to get to work), you can bike commute.

If you have never ridden to your workplace, it helps to make this adjustment to the "just do it" directive: plan and try out your route in advance. Start by mapping your route—by looking at a paper map or using an online map with a bike function—then bike that route on a day that you're *not* going to the office. All maps are not created equal, and this will allow you to figure out the best route without the pressure of needing to make it to the office at a certain time. It will also help you to determine how much time you should allow yourself to get to work; ride at a comfortable pace, and then decide how much time you should allow for your daily commute. Keep in mind that if you're cycling the route on a weekend, the weekday traffic may change how quickly you can get from point A to point B.

What should I wear?

Unlike going out on a weekend ride, when you can happily suit up in sporty clothes and not worry about how sweaty and grimy you will get, when you ride to work it usually means that you will need to arrive in, or change into, a work outfit. Unless, of course, you're a bike messenger or work at a bike shop and can get away with wearing a cycling kit all day.

What you wear is completely dependent on what your commute is like. If you've got thirty miles of rolling hills to cover, you're probably going to want to bring a change of clothes. If you've got two miles of urban streets, you can probably leave the house in your office wear and arrive at the office ready to work. Here's the thing about bike commuting: you can bike commute and look like a normal person. You do not need to invest in an entire wardrobe of fancy gear. That being said, here's some practical advice that will help you.

SAFETY FIRST

When it comes to bike commuting, some of you may not want to hear this, but safety comes before fashion. Especially in the winter months, when chances are your morning commute is in the dark, you don't want to be dressed in your chic all-black outfit. A jacket in a high-visibility color—orange! yellow! maybe even with reflective strips!—is a smart investment for someone who bike commutes regularly.

RAIN WEAR

Any bike commuter, unless they live in a place where rain is a rare occurrence, should invest in good rain wear. You wouldn't want to be called a fair-weather cyclist, would you? No, the two-wheeled life is all about riding no matter the weather. After all, there's no such thing as bad weather, just bad gear.

WATER PROOF BACKPACK

HI-VIS VEST

RAIN PANTS

CUFF GUARD

Invest in a good pair of rain pants that are easy to pull on over your regular pants and shoes (and easy to pull off when you arrive). That means rain pants that zip up a fair length from the cuff. It's nice to have a rain jacket that's a bit longer in the back, as it will keep your torso dry when you are bent over your handlebars. There are plenty of brands out there that make cycling-specific waterproof jackets. This is not the place to skimp on quality; you're buying rain wear to keep 100 percent of the rain off of you, not 60 percent of the rain. Don't be stingy.

Your other best friend in the rain? A set of fenders for your bike. Even if you are suited up in full rain wear and aren't concerned about water splashing on you, a fender helps keep water off your drivetrain. That's good for keeping your bicycle happy.

What if I'm sweaty?

You might get sweaty, and you might not; it all depends on the length of your ride and how hard you ride. Some offices are equipped with showers, which is helpful if you have a long ride to get to work. But for the most part, particularly if you live in an urban area, sweat is probably the least of your worries, so don't let it keep you from commuting.

Some people take the "I'm a bike commuter and I show up a little sweaty" approach, which is to say, they don't care. But if it is a concern, figure out a comfortable biking outfit, and pack your work outfit to change into. You can even bring a little towel, a brush or comb, an extra tube of deodorant, or anything else you may want to use to freshen up. Basically, think of it like the little make-do sponge bath or washcloth shower you rely on when you're camping.

The Essential Commuter Pack

Being a bike commuter is a little easier if you are well prepared. Consider keeping these things on hand in your bag to make the transition from cyclist to worker just a little easier.

WASHCLOTH AND SOAP → While your workplace may not be equipped with showers, a quick face wash before you hit the office can be a game changer.

DEODORANT → If you're into that kind of thing. Also good if you're too lazy to wash.

BABY WIPES → You just might have to change a flat, and in that case, you're going to want to clean off your hands afterward. If you can't wait to get to a sink, baby wipes will save the day.

CHANGE OF UNDERWEAR AND SOCKS → You just never know, especially if you get stuck biking in a downpour. When your feet are soaked, all of a sudden fresh socks are the greatest thing ever invented.

BRUSH → If you have long hair and want to make sure you look presentable for the workday, bring a brush so you can correct any helmet hair.

TREATS → One undeniable side effect of biking to work is that you'll often get ravenous around 10:00 a.m. because you pushed hard on your morning ride. Come to work well prepared with something like Peanut Butter and Chocolate Bars with Apricot (page 143).

How do I ride in a skirt?

For people who enjoy wearing skirts or dresses, or have them as a part of their office wear, this is a dilemma. There is no right way to ride a bike in a skirt or dress; you just have to do what feels comfortable. But for those biking in anything flowing, there are a few ways to make it easier.

Wear leggings or tights underneath → If you have an underlayer on, you won't be worried if your skirt flies up in the wind.

Bring a clothespin → You don't need a high-tech device to keep that skirt from hiking up; you can easily pin it to the underside of your saddle with a clothespin.

Wear a skirt garter → There are special garters out there made specifically for clipping your skirt to the top of your thigh, or you can even make your own.

Sit on your skirt or dress → If you are wearing a longer skirt or dress, pull the front part between your legs and then sit on it, so that you keep it in place while you ride.

Find some loose change → Another secret bike hack? Attach the front and back of your skirt together between your legs with the help of a coin and a rubber band, a strategy popularized by the Penny in Yo' Pants campaign (pennyinyourpants.co.uk). If you don't want the DIY version, they also sell a small device specifically designed for the same purpose.

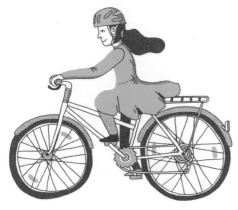

What do I put my stuff in?

Now that we've conquered the clothing aspect of bike commuting, we get to the packing part. Inevitably, you'll have some things you want to take with you to work, and you need someplace to store those things on the way.

BACKPACK

Yes, you can ride with a backpack, and no, you shouldn't feel bad about carrying one. While there are those who will insist that for commuting you need a set of panniers, trust me: a backpack will serve you just fine. And you probably already have one at home, reinforcing the point that you don't need special equipment to become a bike commuter. If you need proof that biking with a backpack is a perfectly acceptable activity, just look at all those bike messengers. The other advantage of carrying your gear in a backpack is that you can use it on any bike and not have to think about your pannier rack setup, which is ideal if you have become so bicycle obsessed that you are regularly rotating through the bikes you ride. Whether you'll want to upgrade from a backpack to panniers will depend on how far your commute is and how heavy your bag is. A longer ride with a backpack stuffed to the brim can become uncomfortable, and in the end, it is all about being comfortable; if you're not, you won't choose to ride.

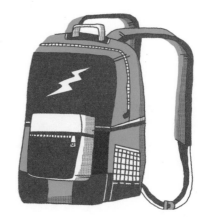

WATERPROOF BACKPACKS

Live in a place where it rains for 70 percent of the year? Get a bag that can withstand that climate. You do not want your laptop or anything else important you have stashed in your bag getting wet. Some backpacks come with a waterproof cover that you can put on; there are also bags made out of 100-percent waterproof material, similar to a dry bag you'd use while camping or boating.

MESSENGER BAG

They are called messenger bags for a reason, and you've probably seen a lot of people ride with them. It's important that the bag be designed to stay in place behind you, often with the help of an additional strap; otherwise you risk having the bag slide around to your front while you're riding, which is both uncomfortable and unsafe if it catches you off guard.

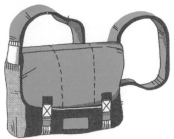

PANNIERS

The benefit of panniers is that they keep weight off your back and shoulders. With panniers, you are letting the bicycle do the heavy lifting. Panniers hang on a rack that sits over your front or back wheel, or both. They tend to have the same shape—sort of a triangle, with a flat section at the top that sits above the bike wheel; the panniers clip into the sides of this flat section and then hang down on either side of the wheel. These can be purchased in any bike or sporting goods shop and can be installed at home, or you can get a bike mechanic to do it for you. Panniers come in a variety of materials; just like with backpacks, consider the weather in which you are going to ride.

STAYING IN GOOD CYCLING SHAPE

What exactly does it mean to be in good cycling shape? It depends on what kind of riding you are doing. A bike commuter and a pro racer are two totally different animals. But let's assume that you're an everyday cyclist, riding your bike to work and maybe doing a few weekend rides here and there.

Let's get one thing straight: being a healthy cyclist is the same as being a healthy human being, and the benefit is that if you are cycling, you are already doing a great job of ensuring that you are getting in physical activity every day. What else comes with being a healthy human being? Eat well. Stay hydrated, and eat your vegetables, please, but don't feel bad about the occasional beer and burger, especially after a long ride!

Simple yoga poses for cyclists

Most people who bicycle a lot forget, however, that while you're getting regular physical activity, it's good to be taking care of your body in other ways. The repetitive motion and fixed posture of cycling can lead to a lot of stiffness and tightness, and an easy way to counteract that is to incorporate a little yoga or stretches into your everyday routine. A yoga practice that focuses on flexibility, core strength, and balance can do you a lot of good when you get back in the saddle. Cyclists are usually particularly in need of hip openers and any type of muscle lengthening exercises. Restorative poses are also helpful, like lying flat on your back and extending your legs straight up against a wall. You can easily do this after you get home from your bike commute; it's a nice way to relax after a day at work and on the bicycle.

CAT/COW

This pose, which is easy to do every morning when you wake up to get you going, helps to lengthen the spine and relieve tension from riding.

Come onto all fours in a "tabletop" position. Focus on your breathing, and as you inhale, lift your head and sit bones to the ceiling, letting your stomach go toward the floor so that there is a concave arch in your back. As you exhale, reverse this arch, drawing your stomach up away from the floor and tilting your head toward the floor.

DOWNWARD FACING DOG

This classic yoga pose helps to lengthen back muscles and hamstrings.

Start on your hands and knees and lift your hips so that you are in an upside-down V shape. Press your palms against the floor and focus on flattening your back. Bend your knees if you need to.

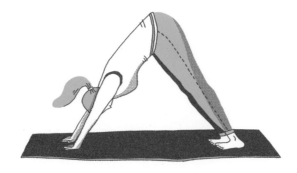

BRIDGE POSE

Release the tension in your lower back and open up your chest with this pose.

Lie flat on your back and bend your knees with your feet flat on the floor. Walk your heels as close to your glutes as possible. Make sure your feet are hip distance apart, then lift your hips off the ground. Roll your shoulders back under your body and clasp your hands underneath your pelvis, then lift your hips a little higher so that your thighs are parallel to the floor. Hold for thirty seconds to one minute.

CAMEL POSE

Ever feel like you get hunched over on the bicycle? This is the pose to counteract that.

Sit on the floor in a kneeling position and extend your toes under your feet so that your feet are flexed. Place your hands on your lower back, with your fingers pointing down toward the floor. Lift your chest upward and let your neck release back to get a supported backbend. If you are a more experienced practitioner of yoga, you can take this further by bringing your hands to your feet, your palms resting on the soles of your feet.

HAPPY BABY POSE

This is an easy restorative pose that feels great after a long ride and is good for loosening those tight hip flexors that cyclists are known for.

Lie on your back and bring both knees to your chest. Hold onto the outside of each foot and spread your knees farther apart, slightly wider than your torso, then bring them down into your armpits. Gently push your feet into your hands at the same time that you use your hands to pull down in order to create some resistance.

CYCLING FOR EXERCISE

One thing that's magical about bicycles is that even if you are not specifically riding one for a sport, whenever you pedal you're still getting in a bit of physical activity. That's why so many people get hooked on bike commuting; not only are you getting to work, but you're getting in a little workout in the process. Our bodies were meant to be active, and bicycles help us do exactly that.

If you're a sports lover, however, you can take your bike riding to a variety of levels.

Road biking

Road cycling is where most people enter the bicycle sports world. That's because all you really need is a bicycle and, well, a road. Here are some other things you may want if you're going to get into road biking:

A ROAD BIKE

If you already have a bicycle and access to a road, then you can go on a road ride. That being said, certain types of bicycles will make this a more enjoyable activity than others. Don't let the type of bicycle that you have stop you from going out on a ride, but if you are looking to do more road riding, then you may want to consider investing in something more than your twenty-year-old single speed.

FRIENDS

While road cycling can be a solitary activity, and some people like it that way, it can be even better if you can get together a group of friends. Don't have friends who ride? It's time to make new ones, with the help of a cycling group. Ask your local bike shop if they organize group rides. There are many bike clubs and organizations all over, which can be a great way to get into the world of cycling.

PORTABLE REPAIR KIT

The beauty of road riding is that you can go anywhere a bike is allowed, far out into the countryside and away from everyday life. But that means that you may not be too close to a bike shop. So bring a patch kit and a portable pump. These are essentials for any road cyclist who isn't being followed by a support vehicle, and they can be life savers.

CLOTHES

There are no absolutes when it comes to what you wear for road cycling; it's all about what you feel comfortable in. Cyclists often wear padded shorts, which add a little extra cushion that makes your backside happier during long miles. A cycling jersey isn't necessary—a T-shirt works well, too—but one nice thing about a jersey is the pockets on the back. Situated so that the pockets are on your lower back when you wear the jersey, this is where you can stash an extra clothing layer, snacks, and some money for that bakery stop.

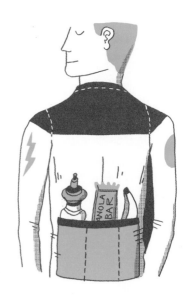

Going on longer rides

At some point, if you like riding a road bike, you may want to get into doing longer miles. After all, the point of being on a bicycle is to ride, and it's amazing how far you can get and how much you can explore simply by using your own power.

But heading out on a sixty-mile ride is a little different from doing a five-mile bike commute. Here are a few things to consider.

TRAINING FOR LONGER MILES

How do you go about training for long rides? There's no right or wrong way, and it all depends on what kind of ride you're doing. But there is one essential to training for any length of ride: time in the saddle. You can be as fit as a marathon runner, but if you haven't spent some time on your bike seat, your butt is going to suffer, the more miles you do. So when planning your training sessions, be sure that you are putting in miles and, in the process, training that rear of yours to get used to the saddle.

PLAN YOUR ROUTE

Serendipity can be a good thing, and some of the best rides are the ones where you just let your wheels guide you, but it's also important to have a general idea of where you are going. Plan your route ahead of time, factoring in which roads are highly trafficked and which ones are not. Remember: the point of a long ride isn't to get somewhere fast, it's to enjoy the journey. This is your chance to take all those scenic routes you have never gotten around to exploring in your four-wheeled vehicle.

CARRY A MAP

In this day and age, it's easy to depend on smartphones and smartphones alone, but if you are riding in an area that you aren't familiar with, it's smart to carry a paper map. No need to carry a lot of extra weight; you can easily make a photocopy of a larger map or atlas and simply carry the section of the map that you need.

CARRY WATER

Running out of water on a ride is simply bad planning. Always carry extra, or know where you can go to refill your bottles.

CARRY SOME FOOD

You don't need to pack a three-course meal, but some snacks are nice. Plus, when you find a scenic outlook you're going to want an excuse to take a break and enjoy the view. Take food that's easy to pack, that you can just stuff into the back pocket of your bike jersey or a small handlebar or under-seat bag.

RIDE LIGHT

Don't be weighed down by nonessentials. Don't bring your entire wallet; grab your ID, a credit card, and a little cash. Don't take your whole wardrobe; if the weather is questionable, take a light extra layer for wind and rain protection.

BE READY TO CHANGE A TIRE

When you're out on the road, you have to be ready to change a flat, because chances are you won't be in proximity to a bike shop, and you probably don't have a support vehicle following you. A spare tube, a patch kit, and a hand bike pump are essentials, and you can't go wrong with some tire levers. And remember: it's much easier to master tire changing at home than on the road, so practice before you head out (see page 71).

Going on organized rides

Bike clubs and organizations put together all kinds of rides. From crazy themed rides to charitable rides, there's something for anyone. Distances will vary, as well as how many people participate, but in general, you can expect the following:

FEES

You're paying for someone else to organize a ride for you. Fees will depend on the type of ride and how many "extras" you get, like a free water bottle or T-shirt. If it's a charitable ride, then part of your donation may be going to the sponsoring organization or foundation.

PREDETERMINED ROUTE

What's great about organized rides is that someone else does all of the route planning for you. Ride organizers work hard to plan good routes, taking into consideration traffic, hills, and how often you need a rest stop to refuel. On an organized ride you will usually be given a route map, and the route is clearly marked along the way, with either arrows painted on the road or signs.

REST STOPS

On larger rides, this fee also pays for pit stops, where you'll usually find plenty of bananas and chocolate chip cookies to keep you happy, even though your butt is sore from all that time in the saddle.

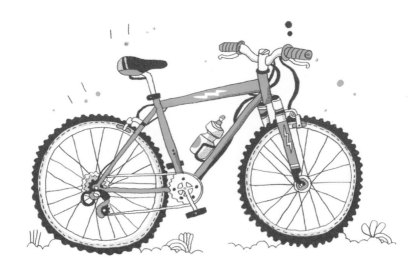

Mountain biking

Mountain biking isn't as accessible as road cycling simply because it's dependent on having access to trails that you can ride on. Urbanites may have to drive a ways to access a trail; rural dwellers may have one right outside their back door.

When it comes to mountain biking, there are different categories.

DIRT JUMPING

Ever seen a video of someone jumping off of huge dirt hills on a bicycle? You know how the neighbor kids spend every afternoon in the forest building a series of jumps? They're aspiring dirt jumping competitors. You'll find that these bikes are similar to BMX bikes, with low seats, and they're made for doing all kinds of fancy tricks.

DOWNHILL

This is the stuff you see on extreme sports channels. Literally going to the top of a hill and riding down it—fast. Without injuring yourself, of course.

CROSS-COUNTRY

Up, down, up and down again. Sort of like the bike version of cross-country skiing. The style of bikes made for cross-country riding is what you will most commonly find in bike shops as well; it's essentially the "classic" version of mountain biking.

SINGLE SPEED

Yes, there are those crazy enough to ride up and down hills on just a single speed—that is to say, with only one gear. Talk to a single-speed mountain biker, though, and they will rave about the simplicity. It's grueling riding, that's for sure, but you never have to think about switching gears.

Cyclocross

Cyclocross sometimes gets put in the mountain bike category, but it's an established enough sport that it deserves its own section. Essentially a cross between road biking and mountain biking, cyclocross is a form of bike racing on bikes with frames that look a little like a road bike's and the knobby tires of mountain bikes, all ridden on muddy trails. Because in cyclocross mud is a good thing, the race season is fall and winter. It's a grimy sport that has developed a cult following, and there are competitions, both amateur and pro, around the world.

There also tends to be a lot of beer and oatmeal involved, and there are often way more spectators than racers, because there are lots of people who like to watch people on bicycles falling in the mud. Just be sure to wear your rain boots if you ever go to watch a race. Things get real muddy.

··

CYCLING WITH CHILDREN

··

There's no reason that biking, whatever kind you are doing, shouldn't be a family affair. Whether you contemplate just a short Saturday trip to the market or you want to plan a long family bike tour, getting the whole family on bikes is just a matter of practice. Nancy Sathre-Vogel of FamilyonBikes.org knows a thing or two about riding with children. She, her husband, and their two sons spent three years cycling from Alaska to Argentina, a total of 17,300 miles. For anyone who has ever thought that bike touring, or just a two-wheeled lifestyle, is for singles only, Sathre-Vogel is proof that enjoying cycling and making it a part of your routine is for everyone, even families with young children. Here are a few of her tips for getting children on bicycles—even for longer tours—and embracing the two-wheeled lifestyle as a family.

Ride—a lot

Nothing is going to get you and your kids used to riding miles like time in the saddle. The more children ride bicycles, the more used to it they get, and when it comes to gearing up for a bike tour or just getting kids into a routine of biking regularly, this is essential.

Start slow

Start with short distances and find a nice comfortable pace. Sometimes with children this can take work, as they are prone to spurts of energy, and often require regular breaks. But teaching them to maintain a constant pace will allow them to ride longer miles. And if you gradually build up miles over time, instead of all of a sudden going on a hundred-mile ride, your child will barely notice the small incremental gains, but he will be building strength all the time.

Make a child sandwich

Not literally, but with your bicycles. Having one adult in front of the child and one adult behind is a great way to teach a child the rules of the road. The adult in front leads the way and sets an example of good riding behavior, while the adult behind can watch the child's back (figuratively and literally). The hardest part for kids to grasp is that they, alone, are in their particular spot in time and space. Just because the leader can safely pull out for a left turn doesn't mean the child can.

Pick interesting destinations

Who doesn't want to ride to go get an ice cream or to go see a movie? Pick interesting destinations so children get excited about riding. Eventually, they'll be so excited about the riding itself that the destination won't matter.

> "Nothing compares to the simple pleasure of riding a bike."
> —JOHN F. KENNEDY

BIKING WHEN TRAVELING

Just as your bicycle is an excellent tool for getting from point A to point B, it can serve the exact same wonderful purpose elsewhere. We're talking about bike travel.

Say the words "bike" and "travel" and most people immediately think of bike touring. We'll get there, but bike touring isn't the only way to incorporate a bicycle into your travels. Even if you are traveling by more conventional methods—airplane, train, and so on—a bicycle can still be an essential component of your trip. So let's take a look at how to incorporate a bicycle into your general travels.

Should I bring my bicycle?

Whether or not to take your bike on a trip will depend on what type of cycling, and how much of it, you are planning on doing. For a weeklong trip in a big city where you just need your bike to get around, renting a bicycle may be a better option than bringing your own with you. But let's say you've booked a cabin in the countryside and you want to have your own bicycle to explore the region. Then you are probably going to want your own set of wheels with you.

TAKING YOUR BICYCLE ON A PLANE

Bikes can easily be checked on airplanes, but that service does come at a cost. Different airlines charge different amounts for checking a bicycle, but in general, the rules for checking them are the same: you'll need to box up your bike.

Bikes can be boxed in both cardboard boxes or, if you're a traveler who regularly takes your bike along with you, a hard-sided box. Packing a bicycle in a box that's appropriate for travel requires taking the bike apart; if you're not comfortable doing that, a bike shop is happy to do it for you at a cost. They'll also have plenty of cardboard bike boxes lying around.

If you want a hard box for your bike but aren't sure if you want to make the investment, ask your local bike shop or bike club. Often they have hard boxes for rent specifically for this purpose.

AVAILABILITY OF BIKE RENTALS AT YOUR DESTINATION

If you want to ride just a few times to explore, then bike rental is probably your safest bet, but you'll want to know what's available before you go. Identify what kind of bike rental programs there are at your travel destination.

RESEARCH WHERE YOU ARE TRAVELING

If you are traveling with your bicycle, chances are at some point you will need to travel on something other than your bicycle, be it from the airport into a city, or from one town to another. Here's where things can get complicated. If your trip requires any kind of public transportation—buses, trains, boats—try to do as much research as you can to find out the logistics of taking your bicycle with you on these modes of transportation. Different countries have different rules and regulations for bikes on trains, for example, and sometimes you need to buy a special ticket in advance if you want to be able to be in the carriage that has space for bike storage.

WHAT ABOUT FOLDING BIKES?

Because of their transportability, some people swear by folding bikes. As these fold down to a smaller footprint, they can be brought inside a building instead of being locked up outside. They are practical for train travel,

Tips for Riding in a New City

GET A (BICYCLE-FRIENDLY) MAP

See if the city you are visiting has a map available that identifies bike paths and bike lanes. This will make exploring much easier. If there aren't any bike-specific maps, take some time to study a general map of the city. Having an idea of approximately where certain landmarks are and getting a general understanding of the city layout is helpful before conquering the streets on two wheels.

PREPARE TO GET LOST

Getting lost is totally fine and nothing to be ashamed of. In fact, it's part of the fun. Just as wandering a city with no predetermined destination can be a great way to explore, allowing yourself to ride without worrying about exactly where you are gives you the chance for travel serendipity. Who knows what you will find? Also, if you are constantly referring to your map while you are riding, you become a safety hazard. Pull over when you need a reference; don't pull the one-hand-on-the-handlebars-one-hand-holding-a-map card. That's a disaster waiting to happen.

BE MORE ALERT THAN USUAL

A new city means new streets, new drivers, and new rules—not to mention, if you're traveling abroad, often a new language, which can make signs much harder to read and understand. All of this makes for a very different cycling routine. Ride more slowly than usual and be extra attentive to your surroundings.

ENJOY THE RIDE

Since you're not going to know the streets, and getting from point A to point B may take a little longer than usual, why not enjoy the process? You are not a bike messenger who needs to speed through traffic; you are an adventurer taking in a new place. Take all the time you need to do it well.

too, as you don't need a train carriage that can accommodate bicycles. Having a night out on the town, and you just can't imagine the ride home? You can fold that bike right up and throw it in the trunk of the taxi. And for the tiny urban apartment dweller, they take up a lot less space than a conventional bicycle. So what are the cons? It's not the preferred vehicle for long or fast rides (although a good option for an around-town bike), some are easier to fold than others, and they aren't always cheap.

Bike share

For another way to bike while traveling, take advantage of bike share. More and more cities are implementing these types of systems, where bicycles are available for use on a short-term basis. You'll find them in cities around the world from Paris to London to New York to Mexico City. Research in advance so that you know how to get a ticket; some machines may not take foreign credit cards, for example, and you will need to buy your ticket online in advance.

Bike share systems may each function a little differently, but the concept is the same: borrow a bicycle to get from point A to point B. Many of these systems have time restrictions, which means you are not taking the same bicycle out for use all day; you are meant to pick one up, ride it to your destination, and drop it off.

When using bike share, remember to check the bicycle before checking it out. Use the *tires, pedals, brakes* method. Check first that the tires are fully pumped, then lift up the back wheel so that you can push down the pedal and see if the crank and chain are in working order. Shift a couple of gears and push the pedal again to make sure that the gears actually work. Test the brakes (both of them!) to make sure that they function. You can also test whether the bell and lights work. Once everything checks out, you're off and running.

BIKE TOURING

Bike touring is about thinking small and simple. It's about getting down to the essentials: you, your bicycle, a few pieces of gear, and some provisions. It's about exploring on two wheels: choosing a destination and getting there by your own power.

If you can ride a bike, then you can go on a bike tour. There is no specific length or type of trip that classifies bike touring; it can be for one day or it can last several years. But there's one thing that all these trips have in common: it's just you, your bike, the road, and your destination(s).

The one assured way to get into bike touring is simply to start. People don't just magically wake up one morning on a bike trip; it all starts with one pedal stroke, just like every other ride. The more

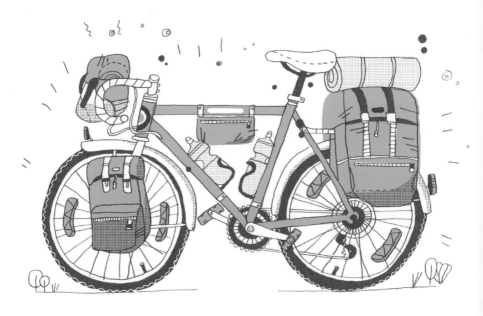

touring you do, the more you will get used to it. Start small and work your way up. Along the way, you just might find that you have a new preferred way of travel.

Five things to get you started on bike touring

Packing everything that you need for a weekend and taking it on your bicycle? For anyone who has never bike toured before, the thought of it may be intimidating. But don't let that stop you. Ellee Thalheimer of cyclingsojourner.com is the perfect advocate for bike touring. She has explored many places by bicycle, from Italy to her home base in the Pacific Northwest, and she is the author of several guidebooks on the topics of bikes and travel. She believes that anyone who can ride a bike can do a bike tour; you just have to be equipped with the right information. Here are her general tips for getting started.

CHOOSE A GOOD TOURING PARTNER

Just because you get along with someone in normal life doesn't mean you're going to get along on a bike tour. Go with someone you don't get annoyed with easily, and before you commit to going, sit down to talk about your expectations and communication styles, as these are crucial to a good bike touring relationship. Talk about what it looks like when one of you gets really tired or hungry, and then how you'd want the other person to deal with that situation. Talking about these things before you go can help to avoid conflict. You still want to like the person after your bike tour is finished, don't you?

BE REALISTIC ABOUT ROUTE PLANNING

When a bike trip is on the horizon, it can be really easy to get excited about doing big mileage. But start easy and allow yourself a relaxing trip that isn't going to push you to the extreme. Beyond miles, also think about elevation; a low-mileage trip with lots of hills isn't the same as a longer but flat ride. If you overshoot on mileage, chances are you won't have fun. The point here is to have fun, not to break any world records. Not up for camping out? Pick a route where you can pop into a B&B. Get used to traveling by bicycle, and you're sure to want to push yourself farther next time.

DON'T GEEK OUT ON GEAR (YET)

For people thinking about bike touring, it seems only natural to start researching bike touring gear online. But start doing a few calculations and you may be quickly put off by the prices. Most people already own gear that will work well—rain gear, helmets, water bottles, etc.—but there are some bike touring specific items that you might need to invest in, discussed on pages 117–119.

BE A MINIMALIST

It may seem like tossing a little thing into your pannier isn't going to make a difference, but if you keep tossing in those little things that you think won't make a difference, pretty soon they will—a *big* difference. Take the opportunity to be a minimalist; think about what your essentials are and what you really need in order to function. And feel free to allow yourself two luxury items: Ellee's are mate tea and a travel hammock.

GET BACK INTO REAL MAPS

Sure, we live in a smartphone world, and these days people are quick to turn to their devices, but in some respects you can't beat the hard copies. They don't break down, you can view the big picture all at once without scrolling around, and if they get wet, they won't die on you. You'll want a good map that has your route clearly mapped, and be sure to bring a couple, in case you forget one along the way.

What kind of a bike do I need for touring?

If you're just starting out, don't feel like you need to go and drop thousands of dollars on an expensive touring bicycle; you want a bicycle that fits you well and that you are comfortable on. Here's the thing: usually, whatever bike you have in your garage is going to be just fine for doing preliminary bike tours. A mountain bike or commuter bike that you can put racks or a trailer on is perfect. Most bicycles (unless you're on a BMX or a tall bike, that is) can be easily adapted to turn into a good touring setup. The important thing is outfitting the bicycle so that you can carry your gear, and that means installing pannier racks (covered shortly).

What about gear?

What gear you need simply depends on what type of bike touring you are doing. A two-day, thirty-mile round-trip at the height of summer is much different from a five-day winter excursion in the snow (yes, people have been known to do that!).

The essentials, of course, are your bicycle, something to carry your gear in, weather-appropriate clothing, a sleeping bag (if you are camping), provisions, and a map. Even if you set out in the middle of summer, on the hottest day of the year, it's also essential to prepare for inclement weather, because you will deeply regret being caught off guard. Remember: there's no such thing as bad weather, just bad gear. This means maybe carrying emergency rain wear, as well as a spare set of socks. Not to mention that you want whatever you are carrying your gear in to be waterproof. The same thing goes for hot days; water and sunscreen, my friend.

Beyond that, some good humor and a sense of adventure will take you far.

Rural Communities Are Great Bicycle Travel Destinations

In 2009, Russ Roca and Laura Crawford of The Path Less Pedaled (pathlesspedaled.com) sold everything they owned to travel by bicycle, pedaling eighteen thousand miles across the United States and New Zealand over the course of three years. Their experiences as travelers informed the work they do now: advocating for bicycle travel as a welcoming, mainstream activity. They actively document and promote the benefit of bike travel to rural communities, for both the local community and the bike traveler. If you're willing to route your trip off the beaten path, you'll often find your way into small communities that you might not otherwise discover. Here are Roca's reasons why rural bike travel is awesome for you and the communities you'll visit.

QUIET ROADS → In rural areas, it's not uncommon to pedal down roads that see only a handful of cars in the course of a day. Here, you don't have to worry about blocking traffic. Instead, you can ramble down blissfully empty country roads—enjoying the quiet, watching the birds, and taking in the otherwise-unseen vistas.

SUPPORTING LOCAL BUSINESSES → Whether it's the diner in town or the taco truck by the campground, you'll get to enjoy the local cuisine, and a small business owner will reap the economic benefits. The same can be said of the local stores, coffee shops, and bars.

COLORFUL HISTORIES → Each small town has a unique character and heritage that makes it different from anyplace else. Taking the time to wander down Main Street or visit the county museum, you can learn about and explore the local history.

REGIONAL TRADITIONS → Besides the experiences awaiting you in the small-town shops, imagine the delight of stumbling onto the annual town parade, crawfish boil, or firefighter pancake breakfast. These events happen regularly in small communities, giving you an opportunity to be a temporary resident and appreciate what life is like there.

NEW CONVERSATIONS → There's something about arriving by bicycle that breaks down the traditional barriers and lets you instantly start chatting with someone from a completely different background. This can be a meaningful opportunity to help break down some of the urban-rural divide.

Once you have decided what you are bringing, you will need something to bring it in. Here are options for transporting your gear:

PANNIERS

Just like for bike commuting, panniers can be used for bike touring; all you have to do is outfit your bike with racks. Remember that panniers are top loaders, which means that it's smart to pack your things in stuff sacks or plastic bags for easy organization.

TRAILER

For longer bike touring trips, when you need to carry more gear, some people opt for a trailer. This can also be great if you are transporting a child, or even your dog—as long as Fido is smart enough to know that he is not allowed to jump out of the trailer when you are pedaling! Of course, trailers can be expensive and certainly add more weight. Most bike tours can be accomplished with a good pannier setup, so whether or not you choose to invest in a trailer will depend on your particular bike tour needs.

PLASTIC BUCKETS

Plastic buckets are an excellent budget-friendly—and waterproof—option for packing. They can be adapted to hang on a bike rack, just as a pannier would; then just pop the lid on to keep your gear covered and ride on your way.

GET CREATIVE

You'll find that in the bike community there's a lot of ingenuity when it comes to packing gear on a bicycle. That can include putting your goods in a stuff sack and using a bungee cord to strap it to the back rack. It can involve sewing your own panniers. It can involve packing as lightly as humanly possible and traveling with barely anything. How you bike tour is up to you, so don't be afraid to experiment a little.

SUPPORT VEHICLE

Laugh all you want, but some people do this. Got a few friends who want to go on a cool trip but won't ride a bicycle? Pack your stuff in their car and have them meet you on the other side. You can rest assured that you will be the one telling the good stories over the campfire.

How do I plan a route?

The easiest bike trips for first-timers are the ones that start from your own doorstep. Unfortunately, not all homes are created equal, and you may feel that you need to get farther away from where you live to start on a good bike tour.

If you are starting a bike tour somewhere other than where you live, the first thing you need to think about is transportation. How are you going to get to your starting point, and how are you going to get back? Can you take public transportation? Do you need to drive a car? If you drive a car, can you park it, or do you need someone to drop you off and pick you up when you are finished?

Because most of us are city people, we often think of a route in terms of being able to access city amenities. We think of a trip as going from one big town to another. The benefit of being on a bicycle, however, is that with the right setup, you can carry all the gear you need for an extended period of time so that you don't have to be anywhere near a metropolis. If you are willing to go off the beaten path, there is a whole world out there to be explored, and what better way to do it than by bicycle?

The Beautiful S240

In the bike world, S240 (pronounced "ess-two-four-oh") stands for sub-24-hour overnight—in other words, a short trip that gets you out on the bike and sleeping somewhere else but back in time to hit work on Monday morning—perfect for the weekend warrior. The term was coined by Grant Petersen of Rivendell Bicycle Works (rivbike.com). For anyone who wants to get into bike camping but may feel a little intimidated by the time and planning commitment of it all, this is a great place to start. All you have to do is pack your bag, get on a bike, pedal to somewhere cool, eat, sleep, and pedal back again. These take much less planning than a longer bike camping tour—it can even be a spontaneous Friday afternoon decision!

PETERSEN'S OFFICIAL S240 PACKING LIST

Sleeping bag

Sleeping pad

Pillow

Tent, for the rain, wind, or bugs

Sleepwear

Headlamp and book

Toothbrush kit

Extra clothing for sitting around camp after the sun sets and it gets cold

Knife

Food and, if you want it hot, a stove

Bowl or plate, and spoon or fork

Bandanas or paper towels for cleanup

These are, of course, the basics; there are other things that you might want to take along, like a camera, a journal, or a travel hammock. What additional clothes you take with you will also depend on where you are going and when. Rain wear might be smart, depending on the elements.

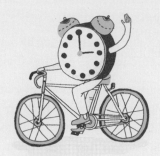

Where to stay

If your bike tour is more than one day, then you will need to overnight somewhere. This can be anything from a hotel or B&B, to a tent, to the barn of a farmer who lets you sleep in it for the night. Where you stay will depend on your comfort level and your budget. If your route passes by hotels or B&Bs, then credit card touring is an option—this means paying for all of your overnight amenities and having a real bed to sleep in. Camping will satisfy your wild side, but also requires bringing a bit more gear—unless you are a true minimalist and sleep under the stars without a sleeping bag (night temperatures permitting).

The important thing about lodging is to think about it in advance, particularly if you are just starting out. Plan out your route so you know where you are staying each night, as well as a backup plan if the shit hits the fan, as it often does. It doesn't work very well to suddenly decide to camp and then realize you don't have a tent or a sleeping bag or a camp stove to boil water for morning coffee.

BIKE CAMPING

Camping while traveling by bicycle is an excellent option if you really want to embrace your freedom. Even camping offers several options.

Tents → You'll want a tent that's as lightweight as possible, but also suited to the seasons that you will be camping in. If you're planning on bike camping mostly in the summer and fall, then you probably don't need a four-season tent. When you're carrying a tent, also consider carrying a little repair kit, just as you do for your bicycle. A spare pole, a stake, and some elastic cord can be incredibly useful in a pinch.

Bivy bags → A bivy bag is a lightweight alternative to a tent. It's a waterproof shell designed to slip over your sleeping bag—in other words, a cozy little cocoon to sleep in. Not the best option if you want to cuddle up at night with your cycling partner, but a smart choice if you're looking to cut weight.

Hammocks → Is there anything better than lying in a hammock after a long day in the saddle? Hammocks may not always be the most practical sleeping option—particularly if you're cycling in a barren landscape with few trees—but in the right situation, they can be a dream come true. As with all bike touring gear, weight is key; do not bring your garden hammock. Opt instead for a camping hammock.

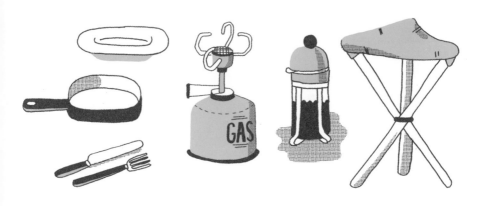

Planning longer trips

Yes, there are people out there who save up their money and then take off for months, even years at a time. This, of course, requires a little more planning than your average weekend trip. And a bit more adapted gear than just your commuter bike with a rack on it. But it's easier to pull off than you may think.

If you think longer tours are up your alley, your best bet is to start on some short ones and work your way up. Plan weekend trips with friends where you escape to a campsite and sit around the campfire and tell stories. Bike to a new city and explore. Pick a place you have always wanted to visit and bring your bicycle. Take a summer off and bike through Europe. See, you're already dreaming of cycling from Alaska to Argentina, aren't you?

Organized bike tours

If you're not up for planning your own bike tour, there are plenty of organized ones, from two-day trips to month-long endeavors. These will cost you, of course, since you get to hand off all the planning and organizing to someone else. If you are going on an organized bike tour, be aware of what will be provided and what won't. Are you staying in accommodations or do you need to bring your sleeping bag? Will there be food? Even if there is food, it's always smart to have your own supply of snacks, because you know what you like, and you know how much of it you want. Plus, when you pull out that bar of dark chocolate, all those other riders are going to want some, and you're going to magically make a whole bunch of new friends.

Eating and drinking

Eating is an essential part of our day when we are *not* on a bike trip, so imagine how important it is when you are clocking many miles a day.

Just as your diet differs from everyone else's, there is no standard Bike Trip Diet that you need to follow. You get to decide what you eat. You can bring all of your own food, or you can plan to eat at restaurants, cafés, bakeries, roadside produce carts, and so on along the way. Or both.

GEAR FOR COOKING YOUR OWN FOOD

If you're bike camping and bringing along your own food, you're going to want to be comfortable with your culinary setup before you go. That means cooking a few meals on your camp stove before you go on your trip so that you know how it works and which utensils, pots, and so on you may need.

Multipurpose is your best friend. As always, you don't want to be lugging your entire house with you on a bike trip. This is the opportunity to be minimal. When it comes to cooking and eating accessories, you want stuff that you can use for a variety of things. This can mean a pot that doubles as a bowl, and a thermos that can be used for drinking hot tea as well as storing leftover soup.

Durability is important. When selecting gear, always choose durability over looks. There is no reason to bring stuff that might break. Chances are you already have a few things in your kitchen that will work; that slightly bent fork is now your camping fork. If you are in the market for some new stuff, choose items that are going to last, and not just for the duration of your trip. Choose titanium, stainless steel, and aluminum over plastic when you can.

THREE ESSENTIAL FOOD TIPS FOR BIKE TOURING

Dan Powell, co-founder of Portland Design Works and Wildeor, is a longtime veteran of the cycling industry and a big-time bike tourer. He recommends the following as bike touring food essentials.

Always carry bite-size snacks and make them easy to reach. Seems like a no-brainer, but jerky, dried fruit, and almonds can be cheap and easy ride foods that will keep you rolling. You never know what you'll feel like eating, so try to pack some choices.

Freeze-dried foods will surprise you. More and more companies are upping the freeze-dried food game. You don't have to settle. Look around and you'll find some delicious choices, like Good To-Go and Patagonia Provisions. Variety is the spice of life, and you don't need to spend an entire trip eating freeze-dried foods when you can explore local restaurants and stores, but it's always smart to travel with at least one or two extra packages of freeze-dried food, just in case. Emergency provisions will ensure that no matter what, you won't go to bed on an empty stomach after a day of long miles.

Take a snack break. On a hot day, when you chance upon some welcome roadside shade, stop and treat yourself to a snack and a cold drink. Take off your helmet and shoes, lean against a tree, and let the world pass you buy for thirty minutes. It'll be awesome.

LET'S TALK ABOUT COFFEE

If you're not a coffee lover, feel free to skip to the next section. If you are a coffee lover, however, pay extra attention. The joy that coffee brings you at home is going to be increased exponentially on a bike trip. There's something about drinking coffee outdoors that is simply unmatched by any other activity. So this is not the time to mess around. You want coffee-making tools with you. I don't mean the espresso machine, but you do want some type of transportable coffee-making device. No, instant coffee will not cut it. Preground will work, and for the true coffee aficionado, whole beans and a hand grinder. You want to be drinking good stuff, don't you?

Coffee-brewing devices. The goal here is something that is lightweight, doesn't create much waste, and gives you the coffee you want. A travel French press is a practical and simple option. The good old paper filter and cone brewer combo is another good option, as long as you make sure that the cone brewer is made from a durable material, and that it fits on whatever cup or thermos you are bringing with you.

OTHER WARM DRINKS

Even if you're not an avid tea drinker, it's so easy to throw a few teabags into your food bag. A decaf or herbal type makes a great end-of-day drink, the ideal thing to send you off to a sleep full of sweet bicycle dreams. Hot chocolate can be another life saver at the end of a rainy day.

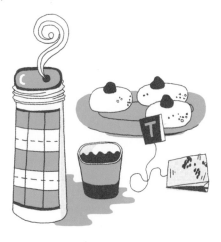

ADULT DRINKS

A little beer and whiskey? Always a good addition to a bike trip if you're a consumer of adult drinks. A stop at a grocery store for an ice-cold beer can break up a long day and even provide a little extra incentive to keep going. Want a little luxury? Carry a flask of your nightcap of choice. You're cycling, so this isn't the time to get blitzed, but it's the perfect time to be enjoying the good things in life.

CLEANUP KIT

No one likes dirty dishes, especially when they're stuck in a pannier all day. Bring some camp soap (the eco-friendly biodegradable stuff) and something to clean with. If you're staying at campgrounds, most often you'll have a water source to wash with.

THE PERFECT MEAL

Spoiler alert: there is no perfect meal. Because what you love to cook and eat may not be what someone else loves to cook and eat. It's all about finding your way to what you love and what keeps you feeling strong on your bicycle. Here are some general guidelines.

Buy food along the way. Not packing food and depending on what you'll find en route? Try to eat smart. Keep your body fueled with good things, but allow for a few treats here and there. When you're staying active, your body will tell you whether it feels good or not with what you're giving it. On tour, you also have the opportunity to explore the local food culture. Grocery stores, as well as local markets, can be full of opportunity for quick and easy snacks that you may never have encountered before.

Invest in good foods. Often a bike trip is the chance to do a budget-friendly adventure. Which means you can feel good about splurging on good food. I'm not talking caviar; I mean good, whole ingredients. An expensive hard cheese that will last a few days and you can eat a few slices at lunch and dinner? Perfect. Crusty bread? Yes, please. Expensive unsweetened dried cranberries from the health foods store? You're on a bike trip; your well-being really does depend on high-quality snacks!

Get foods that can do double duty. Just as you want to bring multi-purpose utensils, you also want multipurpose foods. Things that can work well for both sweet and savory, for breakfast and for dinner. If you are on a trip where you're doing most of your own cooking, make sure that you are carrying ingredients that are good for a variety of meals, and plan out your meals ahead of time so that you are not carrying a bunch of unnecessary extra weight. A bowl of rice or quinoa can be done many different ways, and eaten cold or hot, in the morning, the middle of the day, or the evening.

Bring a spice kit. Spices will save any meal from being boring. Salt, pepper, cinnamon, and chili powder are good ones to start with. Buy small spice bottles at any outdoor outfitter, and pack them in a small bag. Old-fashioned film canisters used to be great for this, if you can find them, but any kind of small sealable containers will do the trick.

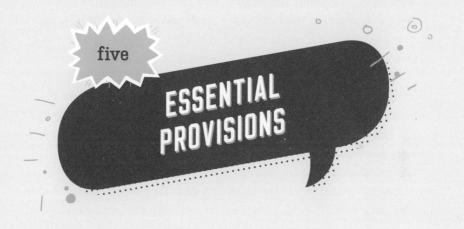

five

ESSENTIAL PROVISIONS

A bicycle doesn't work without someone pedaling it, and to pedal it, you need energy. Fortunately, fueling yourself up for riding is much more interesting than fueling up a car. When it comes to bike fuel, we're talking about food. In fact, your miles per gallon here are way more compelling; think how far you can ride after eating a good breakfast burrito! Just be sure to give your body the time it needs to digest before hopping on the bike.

Some people might say that well-pumped tires, or well-tightened brakes are essential to a good ride. I'd say the real essential is a good meal, because if you're not well fed, that ride isn't going to be half as great as it could be. Food and water are essential to keeping us going on the bicycle—and, while we're at it, in life in general—and because they're essential, why not have a little fun with them?

To be perfectly honest, there's nothing really that special about eating well for a two-wheeled lifestyle. It doesn't require any secret tricks that only cyclists know about. It doesn't take special pills or special drinks. It is exactly like eating healthy in general. In other words, leafy greens, nuts and seeds, and all that other good stuff you know that you should be eating more of. But this type of eating isn't about cutting things out; it's about embracing good food and good ingredients. This chapter is full of ideas for healthy and tasty snacks and meals that will keep any cyclist fueled and happy. Because life is about more than energy bars and gels.

. . . .

STAY HYDRATED

. . . .

Before we can talk about food, we have to talk about water. Water is, after all, much more essential than food. You can ride on an empty stomach, but get dehydrated and you're going to get into big trouble.

If you haven't already, install a water bottle cage on your bicycle. Here you can easily store a water bottle or, on Friday nights, a beer bottle. Mason jars have been known to fit as well, making transporting more entertaining libations quite easy.

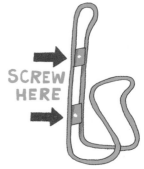

SCREW HERE

Besides water bottle cages, there are also hydration backpacks, with a pocket built to hold a hydration bladder. Hydration bladders are those IV bag–looking things with a tube coming out; they sit against your back in the backpack, and the tube has a valve at the end that clips to your backpack strap on your shoulder and makes drinking as easy as grabbing the end of the tube and putting it in your mouth. These come in a variety of sizes and with a variety of bells and whistles. The important thing to consider is that lighter is better, and if you get a bigger bag, chances are you will fill it up. A few pouches for stashing granola bars, a few bike tools, and maybe a jacket in case it rains are all great, but you don't need to bring your entire pantry and wardrobe with you on your ride. Keep things simple.

If you use a hydration pack, here's one essential piece of advice: keep it clean. There are few things more disgusting than drinking water with a hint of mold. That's easy to avoid as long as you regularly clean your hydration system. Don't let water sit in the hydration bladder for an extended period of time; dump it out every time you are done using it, then give it a quick rinse. Once a week, if you're using it regularly, give it a full wash. Warm water and dishwashing soap will do the trick, but you can also use any of your other preferred home cleaning methods, like vinegar or vinegar and baking soda.

All of this also applies to your water bottles. While it may be tempting to leave the water bottles in the cages when you get home, if they sit in there too long, they can start tasting moldy, so you'll want to dump them out. Right after a ride, however, the water is still good, so either drink up the rest, or water the houseplants with it.

EATING TO FUEL

If there is one thing to remember, it is this: You need real food, and that's that. None of those refined, processed, empty-calorie junk foods so ubiquitous in vending machines and fast-food franchises. Unless you are a professional rider, eating well doesn't have to be a precise science. A well-rounded, balanced diet, full of plenty of vegetables, fruits, lean proteins, whole grains, and nuts and seeds will get you far. Oh, and nut butters. You want the nut butters.

HOW MUCH DO I NEED TO EAT?

Take off for an eighty-mile ride on a Saturday without a few provisions stashed in your pockets, and you are going to be one sad cyclist. You're headed straight for "bonk" land, as it's called in the cycling world. But bonking, or hitting a wall, can be prevented.

How much you need to eat depends on you, just as everyone's usual eating habits differ from person to person. Some people can down five peanut-butter-and-jelly sandwiches on a ride and still want more; others are happy with a few granola bars and a piece of fruit. The only way to figure out your optimal riding food, and the optimal quantity, is to experiment. But in the beginning, better to err on the side of too much than too little. You can always carry extra food that you don't eat, but starving on a ride with nothing left to eat is a more difficult problem to solve.

PRERIDE FOODS

There are differing theories on whether you should eat a huge break-fast or not eat at all. I will say this: ultimately it's up to you. You and you alone can determine what makes you feel best. If you do like to eat before a ride, don't cram yourself full of a huge breakfast fifteen min-utes before leaving the house, because you want to respect your body enough to give it time to digest. If you've got an early morning ride and don't have the time for a leisurely breakfast but are feeling hungry, opt for easily digested foods like smoothies. Really hate eating before you ride? It's okay. Most of us have enough fat stored that our bodies can burn as fuel for a few hours.

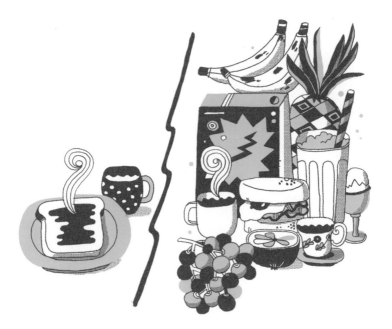

Overnight Raw Buckwheat Porridge

Overnight porridges are the lazy person's breakfast. Or the Not a Morning Person's breakfast. Overnight porridge doesn't require any cooking in the morning; just throw a few ingredients together in a bowl, or jar with lid for easy transport, and when the time is right, dig into your instant breakfast. While overnight porridge is often made with oats, buckwheat is also high in fiber and full of nutrients like manganese, copper, magnesium, phosphorus, and potassium, and gives this porridge a nutty, crunchy consistency. The kind of stuff a healthy cyclist wants to be consuming. In particular, if you're a person who just can't do breakfast in the morning, pop this in a jar with a sealable lid; then you can put it in your bag—or even your water bottle cage—and take it to work with you.

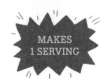

MAKES
1 SERVING

¼ cup (1.5 ounces, 42 grams) raw buckwheat groats

½ cup (120 milliliters) water, for soaking

¼ cup (60 milliliters) dairy or nut milk of your choice

1 teaspoon ground cinnamon

1 teaspoon ground cardamom

Pinch of salt

POTENTIAL TOPPINGS

Yogurt

Fresh or dried fruit

Chopped nuts and/or seeds

Honey

Before you go to bed, place the groats in a bowl with the water and let soak overnight.

In the morning, rinse the soaked groats (they get a bit slimy otherwise). Place the rinsed groats in a bowl or a jar and add the milk, spices, and salt. Add whatever you like, or whatever you have on hand: fresh blueberries, chopped dried apricots, pumpkin seeds, chopped walnuts, and so on. Yogurt will give the porridge a thicker consistency.

Apple and Spinach Breakfast Smoothie

One of the easiest ways to get a breakfast full of good stuff in you is just to cram a bunch of fresh goodies into a blender and press puree. It takes less time than preparing a cooked breakfast, and it's a nice energy-boosting way to start the day. Smoothies can be made from pretty much anything a blender can handle, and you're limited only by your creativity and what's in your refrigerator. This one is heavy on the greens. The almond butter gives it a creamier texture and just a hint of almond flavor. If you're not a fan of almond butter, you can make it without.

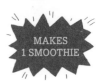

MAKES
1 SMOOTHIE

1 medium-size apple, cored and sliced

A handful of spinach leaves

Freshly squeezed juice of half a lemon

About 1 cup (240 milliliters) water, plus more as needed

2 tablespoons almond butter

Place all ingredients in a blender and puree until smooth. Add more water for a thinner consistency.

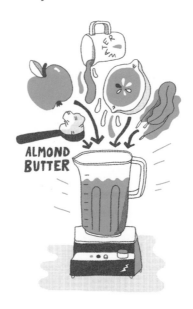

ALMOND BUTTER

Pear Spice Flax Muffins

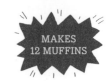

Muffins are an easy breakfast or postride snack. These are made with ground flaxseeds and almond meal, giving them a denser consistency and making them just a little healthier than ordinary flour muffins (and gluten free). Feel free to switch out the pears for other fruit, depending on what's in season. Blueberries and apples work well, too.

MAKES 12 MUFFINS

½ cup (3 ounces, 85 grams) whole flaxseeds, ground fine, or about ¾ cup flax meal

¾ cup (3.5 ounces, 100 grams) raw almonds, ground fine, equal to about 1 cup plus 3 tablespoons almond meal

1 teaspoon baking soda

½ teaspoon salt

2 teaspoons ground cinnamon

1 teaspoon ground cardamom

1 teaspoon ground ginger

2 eggs

⅓ cup (80 milliliters) extra-virgin olive oil

3 tablespoons honey

1 tablespoon apple cider vinegar

1 medium pear, cored and diced

½ cup (3 ounces, 85 grams) raisins (optional)

Preheat the oven to 350°F (175°C). In a bowl, combine all the dry ingredients.

In a separate bowl, whisk the eggs until frothy. Add the olive oil, honey, and vinegar and whisk until well blended. Add the dry ingredients and stir until blended. Fold in the diced pear and the raisins and mix until well blended.

Spoon the batter into 12 silicone muffin baking cups or into a 12-cup muffin tin lined with paper muffin liners. Bake for 25 to 35 minutes, until the muffins are a dark brown. Remove from the oven and let cool in the cups or baking tin.

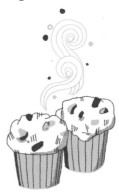

Pantry and Kitchen Essentials for Cyclists

Hannah Grant of hannahgrantcooking.com knows a thing or two about eating well and riding bikes. A chef hailing from Denmark, she's the head chef of a professional racing team and cooks for them out of a truck during major international races. She's the author of *The Grand Tour Cookbook*, a collection of recipes that tells the story of what her team ate during every single stage of the 2012 Tour de France. Here she shares her pantry and kitchen essentials.

COLD-PRESSED EXTRA-VIRGIN OLIVE OIL → Don't be cheap when you buy olive oil; you want the good stuff. Cold-pressed extra-virgin olive oils are full of good fats for your body, and they're easy to absorb and digest, which makes them a great addition to any meal. However, you don't want to be cooking with these high-quality oils; use them in vinaigrettes or just drizzle over your food.

APPLE CIDER VINEGAR → You can make anything taste like heaven with a really good vinaigrette. A little apple cider vinegar, olive oil, and mustard, and you've got yourself a great addition to any meal. Apple cider vinegar is helpful for digestion as well.

CHIA SEEDS → Because of their versatility, chia seeds are a good go-to and can be an integral part of a healthy pantry. Chia seeds' congealing properties work great to add body and binding properties to vegan and gluten-free dishes and baked goods, and they're good in breads, as they help retain moisture.

DIJON MUSTARD → With a good mustard, you can make a tasty vinaigrette, and with a tasty vinaigrette you can spice up essentially anything that's lying around in your refrigerator, which is why this, along with the apple cider vinegar and olive oil, are all in this top five list.

NUTS → Whether they're eaten on their own or turned into nut butter, nuts are incredibly good for you. Grant makes all of her own nut butters, which she encourages people to do. As long as you have a food processor, never again will you have to buy commercial almond butter.

FOODS FOR THE RIDE

For ride food, you want things that will give you an energy boost and are easy to pack. When you are taking food with you on a ride, you have to think about what packs well in a jersey pocket: size, texture, and durability are important. Your best bet is to pack small items and wrap them tightly. Aluminum foil is great for holding wraps and sandwiches together, ensuring that the insides don't ooze out all over the place; ziplock bags are good, too. Keep in mind that, particularly if you are storing stuff in your jersey pocket, you don't want anything that is going to melt. Trail mix with a small amount of dark chocolate is one thing, but milk chocolate bars are prone to melting. However, stopping at a store in the middle of a ride to get an eat-on-the spot meltable treat (I'm thinking ice cream!) is an entirely different matter.

Energy boosters

Packaged bars and gels have become the choice of many cyclists because they're simple to buy, but you don't need chemically fabricated, Technicolor-packaged products to keep you sustained. Nutritious, packable ride foods are easy to make at home.

Carrot Cake Bars

This isn't your average carrot cake. Sweetened with honey, then spiced with cinnamon, cardamom, and ginger, these are the perfect thing to pop into your back jersey pocket or your panniers. You can cut the squares as small as you like, making them easy to transport and stash as a ride snack.

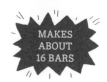

MAKES ABOUT 16 BARS

2 eggs

⅓ cup (80 milliliters) extra-virgin olive oil

¼ cup (60 milliliters) honey

1 tablespoon ground cinnamon

2 teaspoons ground cardamom

2 teaspoons ground ginger

1½ cup (5.25 ounces, 150 grams) finely ground almonds or almond meal

2 cups (6.25 ounces, 180 grams) shredded carrot

Freshly grated zest of 1 orange

¼ cup (1.25 ounces, 35 grams) sesame seeds

Preheat the oven to 350°F (175°C) and prepare an 8 by 8-inch baking pan by greasing or lining with parchment paper. In a bowl, whisk the eggs until frothy. Add the olive oil and honey and whisk until well blended.

Add the spices and ground almonds and mix together. Fold in the carrots, orange zest, and sesame seeds and mix until the batter is well blended.

Pour the batter into the prepared pan and bake for 35 to 45 minutes, until the top is a deep golden brown. Remove from the oven and let cool in the pan. Once cool, cut into 16 equal squares or more smaller squares. Store in an airtight container for up to three days, or for longer in the freezer.

Chocolate Orange Energy Balls

Most power and energy bars are bland and boring. But not when you make them yourself. These use almond butter to hold their shape, and they're easy to carry along on a ride. A warning, though: they are 100-percent addictive.

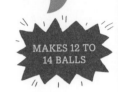

MAKES 12 TO 14 BALLS

½ cup (1.75 ounces, 50 grams) ground flaxseeds or flax meal

2 tablespoons cocoa powder

¼ teaspoon sea salt

1 tablespoon freshly grated orange zest

½ cup (3 ounces, 85 grams) chocolate chips or finely chopped dark chocolate

2 tablespoons honey

½ cup (4.25 ounces, 120 grams) almond butter

½ cup (1.75 ounces, 50 grams) rolled oats

In a bowl, mix together the ground flaxseeds, cocoa powder, and salt. Stir in the orange zest and chocolate chips. Add the honey, almond butter, and oats and mix until well blended.

Scoop small handfuls of the dough and form into balls about the size of walnuts. Store in an airtight container in the refrigerator for up to a week.

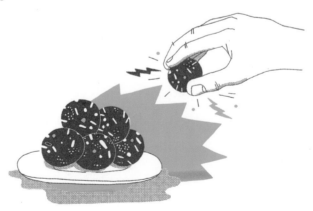

Peanut Butter and Chocolate Bars with Apricot

Peanut butter seems to have almost magical attributes when mixed with eggs; you don't have to add any flour to it to turn it into cookies or bars. Which means we can toss all those complicated recipes. These are all about peanut butter and chocolate, with the addition of chopped dried apricot, and sweetened with honey, keeping you free from processed sugar. These bars are made to be dense; if you want them a little fluffier, add the optional baking soda.

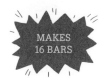

MAKES
16 BARS

2 eggs

¼ cup (60 milliliters) honey

1 cup (9.5 ounces, 270 grams) salted peanut butter (if you use unsalted, just add a little salt to the dough)

2 teaspoons ground cinnamon

½ teaspoon baking soda (optional)

½ cup (3 ounces, 85 grams) chocolate chips or finely chopped dark chocolate

6 dried apricots, chopped

Preheat the oven to 350°F (175°C). In a bowl, whisk the eggs until frothy. Add the honey and mix until well blended. Add the peanut butter, cinnamon, baking soda, chocolate and the chopped apricots. Mix until well blended.

Line a 8 by 8-inch baking dish with parchment paper. Turn the mixture into the pan and using a spatula, evenly spread it out (the mixture is very thick and will not spread out on its own).

Bake for 20 to 25 minutes, until deep golden brown. Remove from the oven and let cool. Cut into 16 equal squares and store in an airtight container. These will keep for three days at room temperature; to keep longer, store in freezer.

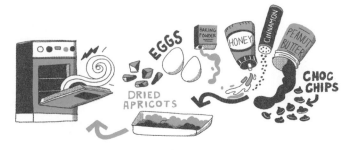

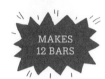

Chocolate Hazelnut Granola Bars

Granola bars are great and all, but what about chocolate granola bars? With chocolate and toasted hazelnuts, and the addition of sweet pieces of figs, these take the granola bar to new heights, and they stash easily for a tasty ride snack. These also work well in bite-size pieces; just cut them into smaller squares. If there are any crumbles left over after cutting the bars, save them and sprinkle over yogurt for a tasty granola topping.

MAKES 12 BARS

1 cup (5 ounces, 140 grams) raw whole hazelnuts

2 cups (7 ounces, 200 grams) rolled oats

¼ cup cocoa powder

½ teaspoon sea salt

½ cup (2.25 ounces, 65 grams) pumpkin seeds

5 dried figs (about 3.5 ounces, 100 grams), finely chopped

⅓ cup (80 milliliters) extra-virgin olive oil

¼ cup (60 milliliters) honey

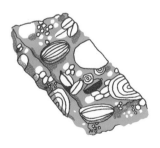

Preheat the oven to 325°F (160°C) and line an 8 by 8-inch pan with parchment paper. Place the hazelnuts on a baking tray and toast for 10 minutes. Remove from the oven and let cool. Place the hazelnuts inside a folded tea towel and roll back and forth to remove the skins. Finely chop the skinned hazelnuts.

In a bowl, mix the oats, cocoa powder, salt, pumpkin seeds, figs, and hazelnuts and stir until well blended.

In a saucepan, combine the olive oil and honey on low heat. As the mixture heats, whisk until it is well blended and thickens.

Pour the oil and honey mixture over the oats and mix together until evenly coated. Turn out the mixture into the prepared pan and press down very firmly, creating an even surface.

Bake for 25 to 30 minutes, until the bars have darkened around the edges. Remove from the oven and let cool completely before cutting into bars; a serrated knife works best. Store in an airtight container for up to one week.

Sandwiches and wraps

Simple sandwiches and wraps are a favorite of cyclists. Just about any spread that works for an ordinary sandwich or wrap will travel well, but spreads that stick the whole thing together without oozing out under pressure are ideal. Here are a few bike-friendly sandwich spreads that will help hold your sandwich or wrap together:

→ Any kind of nut butter (peanut, almond, sunflower, and so on)

→ Hummus

→ Pesto

→ Baba ghanoush

→ Mashed avocado

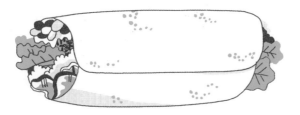

As for sandwich bread, dense bread tends to work the best, as it fares well when it get smashed and compressed into the bottom of your pocket. Sourdough bread has a lower glycemic index, which leads to longer-lasting energy. Tortillas can also be used to make burritos, a cycling favorite. Remember that you're carrying them, though; don't make them too big and overstuffed.

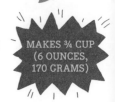

Tahini Pesto

Pesto is traditionally made with pine nuts and Parmesan cheese, but here a little tahini (sesame butter) is used to achieve a creamy consistency that's perfect for bike-friendly sandwiches. Parsley and spinach are the base of this spread, but feel free to switch it out for anything else that's green and leafy: basil, kale, or mint are all tasty variations.

MAKES ¾ CUP (6 OUNCES, 170 GRAMS)

2 cups loosely packed (1 ounce, 30 grams) fresh parsley, well washed

1 large handful spinach, well washed

2 cloves garlic

2 tablespoons tahini

1 tablespoon freshly squeezed lemon juice

¼ cup (60 milliliters) extra-virgin olive oil

Salt

Freshly ground black pepper

In a food processor, pulse the parsley, spinach, and garlic until finely chopped. Add the tahini and lemon juice and pulse a few more times. While the food processor is going, pour in the olive oil, and puree until the pesto reaches the desired consistency. Add more olive oil as needed. Season with salt and pepper to taste. Refrigerate in an airtight container for three to five days.

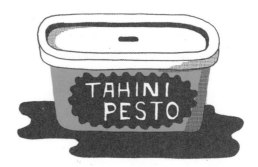

EATING FOR FUN

Isn't all eating fun? It certainly should be. And this is exactly why food and bikes go hand in hand. Whether you're packing for a bike picnic or taking a dish to a potluck dinner, the essential thing about being a food lover and a bike lover is you have to know which foods travel well. And if you really want to transport that slightly travel-unfriendly food, then you need to know how to pack it well.

Bike-friendly foods

If you've committed to a two-wheeled life, then inevitably you're going to start transporting food on your bicycle. When it comes to transporting food on your bike, think small and simple. If you're an avid cook or baker and you start spending a lot of time on a bicycle, you'll find that you will adapt your recipes accordingly. Biking with that triple layered meringue cake with whipped cream? Not so much. But making bite-size meringues, putting some whipped cream in a glass jar with a lid, and then assembling individual whipped cream–topped meringues when you arrive at your destination? Now that's doable.

PACKING FOOD FOR BIKE TRANSPORTATION

Even if you make or buy bike-friendly foods, you still have to transport them. How exactly does one carry food items on a bicycle? Carefully. Some are lucky enough to have a bicycle with a big enough basket to hold a cake pan, or even a cargo tricycle in which they could essentially pack an entire dinner for ten. But let's say you are without said luxuries. If it's just you, your bike, and your carefully prepared food item, here are two ways of transporting it.

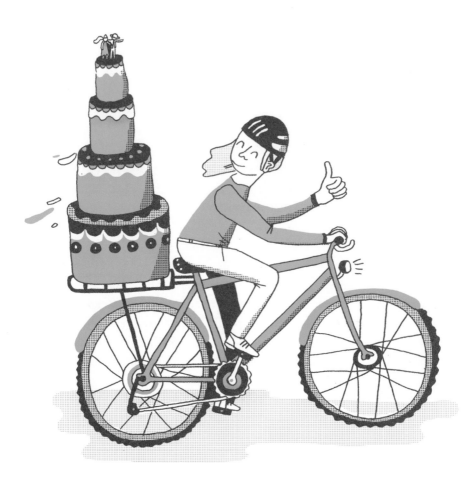

The backpack method. This method requires sealable food containers. After all, no one likes a backpack filled with salad. Recycled glass jars work great, as well as leftover yogurt containers, as long as you are not packing anything liquid. Whatever you are packing your food in, try to make sure that you pack it in your backpack vertically, not sideways or upside down; in other words, with the lid on top. This helps to prevent leakage or an outright food disaster.

The tote bag method. Let's say you bake a cake, and there is no bike basket or pannier or backpack that's ever going to fit it. For that, there's the tote bag method. This can be a bit awkward for first-time cyclists, so make sure you are comfortable on your bike first. Wrap your food item in whatever you deem appropriate, then place it in a tote bag and wrap the tote bag strap several times around one of your handlebars, so that the tote bag doesn't hang too far down and hit the wheel. While you ride, let the tote bag hang from your handlebars, keeping your hand on top of the strap to hold it in place. As you ride and go over bumps, the tote back will swing a little but will provide a little cushion to your precious food item. A much easier ride than bumping along in a bike basket.

Picnics

Is there a greater joy in this world than a bike picnic? No, no there is not. There is literally nothing better than riding on a warm day, stopping and leaning your bicycle against a tree, spreading a blanket out on the ground, pulling out an assortment of food, and eating until you're stuffed. Well, not stuffed to the point that you can't ride home, but almost. Here's what you want to make sure you have in the cyclist's essential picnic pack.

A BLANKET

A blanket is the one thing that sets a *real* picnic apart from just eating outside. A blanket will also double as protection when packing your picnic. You can easily roll a blanket and stuff a wine bottle inside the roll. Instant wine transporter.

A KNIFE

Small, compact, and multipurpose is the way to go. And yes, it needs a corkscrew and bottle opener. Because what is a bicycle picnic without a few drinks?

CUTTING BOARD

Be it for cutting slices of bread or serving a couple of different cheeses, a cutting board is by far one of your best investments. The key is getting one that is durable—you want it to hold up to all that Swiss Army slicing—but lightweight enough that it's not going to weigh you down. Simple wooden boards work well and have that nice rustic picnic look, or opt for a sturdy plastic one.

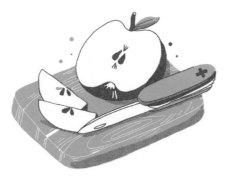

REUSABLE CUTLERY

Don't use disposable plastic forks, knives, and spoons from the picnic section of the grocery store. It's perfectly easy to just bring cutlery from home, or if you want stuff that's specific to your picnic and other outdoor eating adventures, you can invest in a reusable set, in anything from titanium to bamboo.

REUSABLE CUPS

You could just drink out of your water bottle, but for the pleasure of a real picnic, why not invest in a few durable, reusable cups? You can find all kinds—metal, plastic, even food-grade silicone. What you buy is up to you, but remember to consider weight and durability. You want the kind of thing that you can toss into your bag without thinking about it. No point in buying something that's going to break after using it twice.

REUSABLE CONTAINERS WITH SECURE LIDS

Some people repurpose glass jars; others have their grandmother's vintage Tupperware set. Whatever you use to put your food in, first and foremost you want it to do one thing right: keep the food inside. It's an awful feeling to arrive at a picnic site, dismount from your bicycle, get into the food bag, and realize that the salad vinaigrette has gone all over the place. Be sure to think about weight and size, since you will be packing and transporting your containers. You can get reusable containers in a variety of materials. I prefer stainless steel as it's long-lasting and very durable. There might also be containers around the house that you can use, like recycled glass jars or yogurt containers (washed, of course).

A TRASH BAG

You didn't come to the picnic site to dirty it up, now did you? For park picnics, there is usually a garbage can on site, but if you're picnicking anywhere off the beaten track, make sure that you have something with you to collect any rubbish so that you can recycle or dispose of it when you get home.

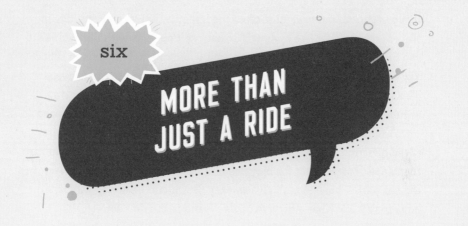

six

MORE THAN JUST A RIDE

Bicycles are not just a mode of transportation or the essential tool for what you do for fun on weekends. The simple machine that is a bicycle is capable of so much more than that. It's a tool for development, a tool for public health, a tool for gender equality, and a tool for building a more sustainable future. The bicycle is full of potential; we just have to use it.

THE BICYCLE AS A TOOL

In a car-centric culture, most often the impetus that leads to trading in two wheels for four has to do with what can't be done with a bicycle that can be done with a car. Grocery shopping, moving, taking kids to school. Yet all these activities can and do take place with the use of a bicycle. This is not an argument for ditching your car immediately, but it is an argument for thinking more creatively about how a bicycle can be used.

A bicycle can be a workhorse if you want it to be. Certainly there is the question of infrastructure; unfortunately, most of us live in places that were designed not for bicycles, but for cars, and as such, replacing the car with a bicycle isn't always easy. But it can be done. We just have to rethink what a bicycle can do—and it can do a lot.

Cargo bikes

Cargo bikes come in all shapes and sizes and can be used for a variety of purposes. If you want to pedal the kids to school, there's a bicycle for that. If you want to move heavy equipment, there's a bicycle for that, too.

One city that embraces bikes as tools to everyday life is Amsterdam. Spend a weekend walking the streets of this bike-centric capital, and you will inevitably see a few toddlers, and maybe even a dog, crammed into the front of a cargo bike—the eco-friendly version of the minivan. But around the world, people are using bikes to haul things around. Nowadays, it's not uncommon in big cities like New York City to see a person pedaling a delivery bicycle, maybe for a restaurant that uses pedal-powered delivery service; it's a lower-impact way of doing urban deliveries, keeping trucks off of already-clogged streets. In urban areas, cargo bikes are a smart investment for companies—it's why

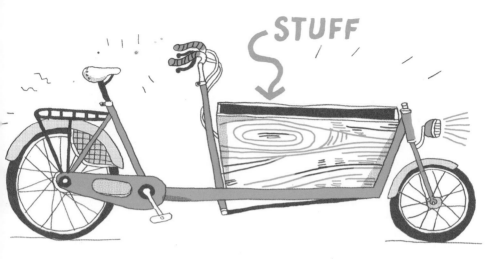

companies like DHL and UPS have tested cargo bikes and electric assist delivery bikes in various European cities. They cost less up front, they reduce traffic congestion, and the company doesn't need big loading docks to load and unload their goods.

Compared to a car, the cargo bike is inherently low tech; it doesn't need gas, it's not responsible for emissions, and it won't get you stuck in a traffic jam. You don't even need a license to drive it. While it may seem daunting to transport things that you might otherwise use a car for, the important thing to remember with using a bike for cargo is that you are letting the bicycle do all the work; all you have to do is pedal, shift, steer. This is all about utility cycling. The following are some of the main types of cargo bikes.

CARGO TRICYCLE

This traditional Dutch cargo tricycle, called a *bakfiets*, is what most people think of when they hear the term *cargo bike*. These have a longer wheelbase in the front to accommodate a box, which is where the word *bakfiets* comes from in the first place: it means box bike. Into this box, you pop your kids, your groceries, your new chair that you just bought—whatever it is that you need to cart around. Beyond the traditional *bakfiets* style, there are also cargo tricycles that are built to have a cargo space on the back of the bicycle.

LONGTAIL BICYCLES

A longtail bicycle is intended for people that want the advantages of hauling a trailer without actually hauling a trailer. You get around the issue of having a trailer by extending the rear of the bicycle. Xtracycle is a brand that has made this style of utility bicycle famous. You'll see longtail bicycles with everything from groceries to passengers—yes, even multiple children—sitting on the back.

CYCLE TRUCK

Cycle trucks can't carry as much gear as a cargo tricycle or longtail, but they are also lighter, which makes them a good midrange cargo bike. This bicycle typically has a rack attached to the front of the frame, as well as a smaller front wheel to deal with the rack's lower center of gravity. This isn't a new and modern thing; Schwinn actually put a cycle truck into production back in 1936.

EVERYTHING ELSE

Start looking around, and you'll see all kinds of utility bicycles. Got an old used bicycle that you want to play around with? If you want to convert your bicycle into something more utilitarian, there are plenty of DIY guides out there. In the market to buy a cargo bike? It's exactly the same process as for buying any other kind of bike; think about exactly what you want it for, what you're going to be carrying, how much, and so on. There's a cargo bike out there for everyone.

What to do with a cargo bicycle

Cargo bicycles can serve many purposes. They're the workhorses of the bicycle world. Think outside the box. Bicycles aren't just for riding from point A to point B. We see them as limited in what they can do mostly because we think of them for only one purpose. But if ever there was a multipurpose vehicle, the bicycle, particularly a utility bicycle, is definitely it.

GROCERY SHOPPING

If you shop regularly in small quantities, you don't need a cargo bike to get your groceries home; your average bike will do just fine. If you like to shop less often and stock up when there's a sale, a cargo bike can definitely make this task easier. In fact, having a longtail bicycle—or even just a bike with a better basket setup, like a cycle truck—just might make you more inclined to take your bicycle to the grocery store.

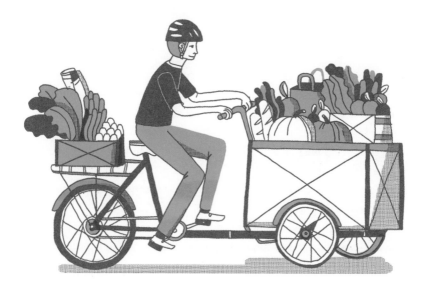

CARRY SPORTS EQUIPMENT

Cycling around with a surfboard may sound like the most ridiculous of endeavors, but it's totally doable. Some companies build special setups so that you can carry your surfboard, or even your kayak, on the side of your bike, and there are plenty of people who retrofit their own bicycles to do the same thing.

TRANSPORT PEOPLE

You can put a child's seat on any normal bicycle, but with a cargo bike you can carry much more weight, which means that it's not just toddlers who are going to have all the fun. An adult passenger can easily sit on the back of a longtail bicycle or in the front of a cargo tricycle.

BUILD SOMETHING

With the right cargo bike setup, you can easily cart around building tools and supplies. Whoever said that a construction site had to be filled with big trucks?

MOVE

This can seem like a daunting task to a first-time cyclist, but there are people out there who do entire moves by bicycle. Yes, packing up an entire house and moving all their stuff on two wheels. Moving by bicycle is a feasible option when you are moving somewhere within the same town, and particularly if you have a few friends with cargo bikes or bike trailers. It's always better to make a group effort out of it; just be sure to promise some cold beer and pizza at the end of it to turn it into a bike move party.

Coordinating longer moves is possible as well, as long as you put time into planning the route, getting a devoted group of friends to help you move, and being smart about packing up your stuff. Don't want to do the work yourself? There are even moving companies out there, from New Orleans to Montreal, that operate 100 percent by bicycle or offer bicycle moving as an option.

THE BICYCLE AS A BUSINESS

If you have fallen madly and passionately in love with bicycles and cycling, an easy outlet for that love is a bike shop. But a bike shop isn't the only way to combine bikes and business. Nowadays, particularly in urban areas, bikes are playing a central role in anything that requires a business to be mobile.

An obvious one is food; we're talking food bikes instead of food trucks. From taco trikes to mobile espresso bars, bicycles are empowering food business owners to get around in a more sustainable manner. And also, isn't it more fun to buy your lunch or coffee from a bicycle?

Bike cafes

For some reason, bicycles and coffee are a perfect match. Think of a bicycle ride that ends at a café with a cup of coffee and a treat. Around the world, coffee entrepreneurs are incorporating bicycles into their business, be it with mobile coffee carts or delivering freshly roasted coffee by bicycles to retailers and other coffee shops, like Bicycle Coffee in Oakland, California, Conduit Coffee in Seattle, Washington, and The Coffee Ride in Boulder, Colorado. In Sweden, there is even a budding global franchise of mobile cafés: a company called Wheely's is allowing aspiring business owners to buy one of their bike café setups, and since they started, they have positioned over thirty cafés in ten different countries.

Vending cart bikes

Forget the ice cream truck. Imagine spending your summer cycling around a neighborhood selling sweet, cold treats. As long as you can outfit your bicycle with a freezer chest, you can start a mobile ice cream business. And that's just the beginning for mobile vending carts. Cinnamon rolls, hot dogs, tacos; you name it, and someone is probably selling it out of a vending cart bicycle. And if they're not, maybe you should start one. Nowadays there are also companies producing and selling this style of mobile vending cart, which makes launching a pedal-powered business all the more easy.

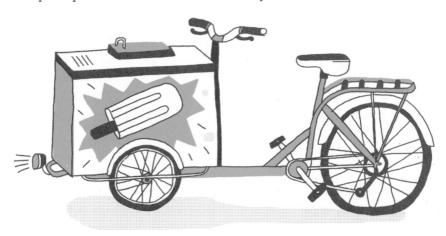

Food delivery

While bicycles can operate similar to food trucks, and prepare the food on site, they can also be used to deliver food, from restaurants, grocery stores, or any kind of independent food business. From sandwiches to gluten-free pastries, bicycle delivery can definitely have a sweet side.

Pedal-powered farm to table

With the rise in popularity of community supported agriculture (CSA), it would make sense that bikes would naturally make their way into the equation. Urban farms in particular are the perfect candidates for delivery by bicycle, allowing CSA members to know not only that their food is grown locally, but also that it's delivered in an eco-friendly manner.

. . . .

THE BICYCLE AS A CHANGEMAKER

. . . .

Bicycles can change the world! That may come off as a bold statement, but there was certainly a time when bicycles sparked a revolution. They were instrumental in the late 1800s and early 1900s in improving road quality. A bicycle didn't need to be fed, like a horse. And you didn't need to maintain a carriage. Or have any land to keep all of those horses that helped you get around. A bicycle was freeing. It was a new and democratized form of transportation.

Bicycles helped fuel the women's rights revolution, an essential part of the women's suffrage movement. "To men, the bicycle in the beginning was merely a new toy, another machine added to the long list of devices they knew in their work and play. To women, it was a steed upon which they rode into a new world," wrote a journalist in *Munsey's Magazine* in 1896.

The bicycle meant that women could get out and about and socialize on their own. It also meant that the definitions of femininity changed. Think of women's clothing of the Victorian age. Not so bike friendly. And so bloomers came to be, and later, pants. At the time, they were considered an abomination by some, but nowadays we take them very much for granted. "The woman on the wheel is altogether a novelty, and is essentially a product of the last decade of the century," wrote a journalist in *The Columbian* in 1895. "She is riding to greater freedom, to a nearer equality with man, to the habit of taking care of herself, and to new views on the subject of clothes philosophy."

Nowadays a bicycle seems like such a simple thing that we often forget how revolutionary its role has been. The bicycle is in fact a vehicle for independence and change, and that continues to be true around the world. In terms of women's rights, the bicycle provides freedom of mobility, an essential component of equal rights; when a woman can get from point A to point B by her own means, this can be life changing. In the Middle East, women's cycling groups from Cairo to Kabul are slowly changing gender perceptions. Bicycles can also be a crucial tool for development, used to increase access to schools and health care. Changing lives isn't always complicated; it, too, can be as simple as giving the gift of two wheels. In Africa, organizations like World Bicycle Relief work to provide bicycles to health workers so that they can cover more ground in a day. In countries like Cambodia and India, organizations work to provide girls with bicycles so that they can get themselves to school, and in turn get an education, perhaps the most meaningful investment in terms of development.

"One child, one teacher, one pen, and one book can change the world." That was the message delivered to the United Nations by Malala Yousafzai, the Pakistani advocate for education and women's rights, as well as the youngest-ever Nobel Prize laureate. What if we also added "one bicycle"? Think of what a bicycle does in your community. Now imagine what it can do in a developing community. A bicycle can allow a child to go to school; it can allow access to health care. It can simply serve the purpose of introducing fun and joy to a dismal routine. We may not solve all the world's problems with bicycles, but we might start better dealing with a significant amount of them.

While the bicycle may not at first glance seem revolutionary, let us not forget its power. And to harness that power, there's one thing that we can all do: ride. Let's be a part of the two-wheeled revolution. Maybe it's a ride to the grocery store, or maybe it's a month-long two-wheeled adventure. Whatever we make of them, more bicycles are a good thing. Let us embrace the two-wheeled life and ride into the future as happy, independent, and free human beings. The more we pedal, the farther we go.

Does this mean you are an activist now?

Bike activism. Just mention these two words and it sounds like you're talking about a very specific, devoted group of people. Well, you know what? If you ride a bike, you are a bike activist. Certainly, there are different levels of bike activism, but the truth is that the simple act of choosing to ride your bicycle is an action that speaks louder than words. Getting on your bicycle and leading by example makes you part of the bicycle revolution, whether you know it or not. And as long as you are part of it, you may as well find out more about it.

As you get more and more into the bike movement, you may feel yourself wanting to take part in new and different ways. There are a variety of organizations out there that could use your help (see Resources, page 176), be it financial or volunteering, and if you want to be more active in the overall cycling community, these can be a great place to start.

Here are some other ways to advocate for cycling:

RIDING MORE

The more cyclists out there, the better. A revolution is all about helping that revolution move forward, and by simply getting on a bicycle, you are doing just that. We can all do more, no matter what cycling level we are at. Maybe it's bike commuting to work one more day a week, or maybe it's committing to cycling even when the weather is nasty. Or maybe it's challenging yourself to take part in a cyclocross race. Whatever it may be, the more you ride, the more power you add to the overall bike revolution.

ORGANIZING RIDES

You don't need to be an official bike tour organizer to plan a ride. Put together a fun route and invite a few friends who are new to cycling. Plan a picnic and bring a bottle of bubbles and some cookies along as some good enticement to pedal all those miles. Or get up early and end the ride at a coffee shop. The more people we get on bikes, the better, and if you have to bribe your friends a little bit to do just that, it's totally fine.

GETTING EDUCATED

As crazy as it may sound, there's an antibike lobby out there. There are people who argue against better bike policy, against more bike lanes, and against general pedestrian and cyclist safety. The best way to go up against that? Arm yourself with knowledge. Organizations out there like People for Bikes work hard to compile statistics on bicycling (peopleforbikes.org/statistics), and if you start to get to know the literature, then you'll be better equipped to get into the more bikes versus fewer bikes arguments.

STARTING A TWO-WHEELED PROJECT

Bicycles are capable of a lot, and they have plenty of uses outside of the familiar ones. Come up with a creative way to use a bicycle. Maybe you partner with a local business to help them do bike deliveries; maybe you retrofit your bicycle to be able to make pedal-powered smoothies; or maybe you do like the Feminist Library on Wheels in Los Angeles, and cart around books via bicycle.

How to Organize a Bike Ride

It's fun to ride with other people, and you don't need to wait until the right organized ride comes along. You can plan your own. Be it a cross-town ride that ends at the local microbrewery or a Saturday jaunt out into the countryside, you're free to organize any type of ride you want. Remember that if you are organizing a ride, the riders are going to hold you responsible—for their safety, and for their entertainment. Good planning will lead to a good ride, and ideally leave your riders inspired to bike more in the future.

CHOOSE A ROUTE

Route planning is essential when planning a ride. Know the roads and the route, how much traffic to expect, and what safety precautions you may need to take. Also take into consideration the day and time you are planning to ride. Ride the route yourself before you go so that you know it well.

CHOOSE A THEME

A good way to think about planning a ride is to think about a theme. Maybe you want to explore local food spots—a weekend ride to check out artisan cheese makers and vineyards, perhaps—or maybe you want to share all the secrets about your city—an urban street art tour, let's say. Whatever your theme is, be sure you're knowledgeable about it. Your riders are looking to you for all of their information.

COSTUMES?

This doesn't work for all rides, but who doesn't love a good excuse to dress up? Costume themes can make an average bike ride an awesome bike ride. Superhero Bike Gang, anyone?

TELL RIDERS WHAT THEY NEED TO BRING

Is this a long ride where people might want to bring along snacks? Will you be riding after dark, so riders will need their lights? Should they bring cash for buying produce at the farm you're visiting? Don't assume your participants know what to bring; provide them with an easy checklist.

CITIES AND BICYCLES

It's not just individuals who are pushing for more bikes; cities around the world are catching on to the fact that investing in cycling infrastructure is a good thing. It helps with citizens' health, promotes small businesses, and makes cities cleaner and less congested.

Car-free days

Many cities around the world have begun to institute car-free days—designated days when certain streets are free from motorized traffic. In other words: a cyclist's dream world. Bogota, Colombia, is credited with pioneering the concept, shutting off certain main roads every single Sunday. Referred to as *ciclovía*, which in Spanish means "cycleway," this type of initiative has taken off in many other places. There is an entire network called Ciclovías Recreativas de las Américas (cicloviasrecreativas.org). The organization advocates to get more cities implementing similar programs, to promote not only cycling, but healthier communities as well, and they maintain a map to show all of the *ciclovías* in both North and South America.

Bike to Work Day

To support bike commuting, as a part of National Bike Month in the United States, sponsored by the League of American Bicyclists each May, there is also a National Bike to Work Week. Many cities and local bike organizations participate, and they often organize their own Bike to Work days to promote more people commuting to work on two wheels. But remember this: Bike to Work Day is kind of like Earth Day;

it's great to devote a whole day to being excited about bike commuting, but it's something that more of us should be doing the other 364 days of the year as well.

Bike parking

If you have a hard time parking a bike safely and securely, chances are you won't be as willing to ride. Investing in bike parking is a smart move on the part of city planners; think of how many bikes you can fit into an average car parking space. There are innovative bike parking systems around the world, like the underground bike parking in Japan where bicycles are fed into a parking station and then taken into an underground well and parked, keeping the bicycles off the street and leaving more space as well as keeping them protected. To encourage more people to ride bikes, and in turn help ease the pains of car parking, in some cities you'll find bike valets at events, from farmer's markets to baseball games. Unlike using a car valet, however, bike valet service is often free. Planning your own event? Why not offer a bike valet?

Incorporating bicycles into public transportation systems

In Europe, there's currently a project called Bike-Train-Bike; taking inspiration from the Dutch system, it is implementing projects across Europe that focus on promoting the combination of bikes and trains as transportation as opposed to cars and trains. You may not be willing to bike fifty miles to work, but imagine if you had a three-mile ride to a train station where you could easily park your bike and then take the train the rest of the way? While the train infrastructure isn't as developed in the United States as in Europe, imagine if every park-and-ride was a bike-park-and-ride, with better infrastructure in place to encourage people to bike to the bus station. This intermodal transportation is definitely a way of creating a more sustainable future.

Building better bike lanes

When it comes to bike lanes, if you build it, the cyclists will come. We cyclists want to feel safe; we want to ride and not fear for our lives. A 2012 study by researchers at Rutgers that looked at various data sets from ninety different U.S. cities concluded that "cities with a greater supply of bike paths and lanes have significantly higher bike commute rates." The Green Lane Project is one initiative to help cities build better bike lanes, and there are organizations around the world that work hard to make this a priority for urban planners.

Of course, in the United States, advocating for bicycles often causes an uproar. Why? Because it challenges the status quo of cars in our car-centric culture.

. . . .

ARE PEOPLE REALLY AGAINST BICYCLES?

. . . .

Once you've discovered the love of two wheels, it seems downright crazy that anyone would be against bicycles. But they are out there. Whether it be campaigning against a new bike lane or challenging bicycle safety laws implemented by cities or even threatening (or dealing out) physical abuse of bicyclists while riding, there are a fair number of people who aren't so bike friendly. Some of this isn't vicious; it simply reflects a stigmatizing attitude toward cycling that we have to work hard to change. In a car culture, cycling is often seen as the silly option that you choose only if you can't afford that rite of passage to adulthood, your own car. In some communities, if a person is on a bicycle, they are assumed to be poor, with not enough money to own a car, or worse yet, a drunkard who has lost their license and is now forced to use two wheels to get around. There are plenty of stories of cyclists having things thrown at them or simply being verbally abused while on the road. Some people even joke about hitting cyclists, as if it were a fun pastime.

How do we change this? We continue to be advocates for change. Cyclists have a right to the road. If you choose to ride a bicycle rather than drive a car, you should feel empowered to do so. The most fundamental thing that we can do to change the cultural prejudice against cycling is to continue riding and continue having conversations. Cyclists are normal people, functioning members of society. We do not deserve to be treated like second-class citizens. And if we want to take the car lane once in a while because it makes us safer, then we will do it. Unfortunately, that may be seen by the car culture as an extreme, annoying act, which escalates this ongoing battle between cyclists and drivers.

I say this not to further fuel the conflict, but to remind us all that we shouldn't allow this unfortunate situation to silence us. History has shown us that changing the status quo isn't easy. It's often downright difficult. It takes revolutionaries. But fortunately, for the most part being on a bicycle doesn't feel like being a revolutionary. Ask most people why they ride, and they will probably launch into a long explanation of how great it makes them feel, physically and emotionally. I don't ride because I want to make a statement. I ride simply because I want to ride.

How to counter the top myths about cycling

There are all kinds of arguments against cycling out there. Elly Blue has written on this topic for a long time; she is the author of *Everyday Bicycling: How to Ride a Bike for Transportation* and *Bikeonomics: How Bicycling Can Save the Economy*. She speaks regularly at bike conferences around the world about bike policy and more. She is well versed in the arguments that cyclists often face, and she is happy to help you counter them.

MYTH: BIKES DON'T PAY FOR THE ROADS

In the United States, the road system was originally intended to be funded only by taxes on gas and various car parts like tires. But the cost of building and maintaining enough pavement for everyone who wants to drive (and park) their car is so astronomically high that gas tax covers only about half of it. So if you ride a bicycle instead of driving a car or taking public transportation, you're still paying for the roads through your general taxes—actually, you're subsidizing the car drivers' driving habit.

MYTH: BIKES SLOW DOWN TRAFFIC AND CAUSE POLLUTION

When you're driving a car capable of going 120 mph, on a road with a 25 or 30 or 35mph speed limit, and you're stuck behind a bicyclist traveling at 15 mph or less, it can feel unbelievably frustrating. But what is actually causing you to burn excess fuel isn't needing to go at pedaling speed for three blocks during your commute—it's hitting the gas to try to get ahead, only to come to a screeching halt at the next light, rinse, repeat. If everyone drove at a slower, steadier rate—in downtown areas, about as fast as a bicyclist can go is optimal—everyone would get where they're going much more quickly and generate less pollution.

MYTH: THERE ISN'T ENOUGH SPACE ON THE ROAD FOR BIKE LANES

Someone driving a two-ton car with the footprint of an efficiency apartment is always going to feel like there isn't enough space on the road. This problem, however, is caused not by bike lanes, sidewalks, buildings, or the person you saw yesterday biking up the street the wrong way. Researcher Peter Jacobsen has a great analogy to describe this sense of scarcity. We tend to think of traffic like a river, one that will flow more freely the wider its channel—that is, the more car lanes you add to the highway. But actually, says Jacobsen, traffic behaves like a gas, expanding to fill whatever space is available. So when you reduce the number of lanes dedicated to cars only, people drive less. And when you add to the amount of space designated for bicycles, bike traffic will grow to fill that space. Of course, if all traffic went at a more reasonable speed, we wouldn't need nearly as many bike lanes.

MYTH: BICYCLING ISN'T SAFE

The first assumption in this myth is that other ways of getting around— like walking, taking the bus, and especially driving—are totally safe. The reality is that none of these are completely safe because roads are built to encourage fast driving, not safe driving. Statistics change daily, but every year tens of thousand of people die in car crashes in the United States, and millions are injured. Bicycling has another great safety advantage over driving—you are safer from the numerous medical problems caused and exacerbated by prolonged stationary sitting, combined with the extreme stress of driving in traffic. Both stationary sitting and stress are shown to shorten your life span well beyond the risk of being injured in a crash. While you're sure to encounter stressful situations on your bicycle, you'll work them off immediately. In a car, you can only continue to sit and stew over whatever is bothering you.

All bicyclists run red lights! So goes the myth. *They don't care about safety! They think they're above the law!* There's more than a small element of confirmation bias in this mindset. There is some partial support for one accusation: Many people on bikes in cities around the world can be seen rolling through a stop sign, dashing through a red light, or cruising the wrong way down a one-way street. This isn't because we're a lawless breed, though—it's typically because road design and driver behavior create a hazardous situation that makes it often seem safer not to stop in front of a hurtling taxi as the light turns red, or to take a shorter, wrong-way route rather than risking

Getting Together with Other Cyclists: Critical Mass

Ever heard of Critical Mass? Chances are if you live in an urban area, you may have already come across this term. It refers to a mass bicycle ride, most often taking place on the last Friday of each month in cities around the world. It's not much more complicated than that; just people gathering together with their bikes and riding around, free of charge and open to everyone.

The event originated in San Francisco in 1992 and since then has spread to cities around the world, encouraging mass citizen mobilization. Of course, because of this, many have taken to seeing Critical Mass as a political statement, and more of a protest than a ride. Many organizers and participants, however, insist on the celebratory and spontaneous nature of these gatherings; it's actually just people who love bicycles coming together to ride, and for a short moment, feeling like they outnumber cars. Ultimately, the participants take part in Critical Mass for different reasons, but there's no denying that they have played a major role in galvanizing urban cycling culture.

three left turns on busy arterials to go with traffic. The real clincher: When Chicago put separated bicycle lanes all over their downtown core, a study found that while previously only 31 percent of cyclists had waited for red lights, with the new bike infrastructure 81 percent waited. In bike-friendly Portland, Oregon, a study found that 94 percent of cyclists wait at red lights. Meanwhile, a U.S. government survey found that 56 percent of drivers admit to running red lights, and two people a day die in the United States because of this.

WHEN CAN YOU CALL YOURSELF A CYCLIST?

What is it that truly defines a cyclist? Do you have to ride a certain number of miles a week? Do you have to own a certain number of bicycles? Do you have to have special shorts? Do you have to go on organized rides?

Being a cyclist doesn't have to include any of these. Simply put, a cyclist is someone who loves to ride a bicycle. You do not need to be a professional racer; you do not have to go on hundred-mile rides on weekends. You do not have to drink protein shakes before 5 a.m. rides; you do not have to know what every single part on your bicycle is called. If you have committed to riding your bicycle, and you have fallen in love with it in the process, then you are one who cycles, and hence you may call yourself a cyclist.

I say this because so often people are intimidated by the bike world. I myself have been there. I once sat in a room full of women, all involved in the bike industry in some way—be it racing, owning a bike business, or just advocating for bicycles. "Well, I'm not really a cyclist,"

I said, trying to think about the last time I had gone on a long weekend ride and feeling sort of guilty for not challenging myself to sign up for cyclocross season. "But I do like to ride, and I bike every day," I added, in an attempt to justify myself, moderately intimidated by the group of bike-savvy people around me.

"Well, then, of course you *are* a cyclist," said one of them.

This has stuck with me through the years, and I say it as a reminder that there is no one activity that all of a sudden makes you a cyclist. Some may race and never bike commute. Some bike commuters may never choose to get on a road bike.

But there is no need to discredit ourselves and make excuses based on what we do or don't do. We shouldn't feel that we are not skilled enough, haven't ridden enough miles, don't have the right kind of bicycle. On the contrary, we should feel empowered. Empowered to learn more, explore more. A love of cycling is enough. A desire to get on a bicycle every day (well, most every day). A need to feel the wind on your face as you ride down a hill. This is all you need to call yourself a cyclist.

A cyclist is a person who loves to ride a bicycle. End of story. You never know where that love will lead. Maybe one day you will take off on a month-long bike tour; maybe you will commit to commuting every day; maybe you will petition your local town to install bike lanes. But for now, that love and passion for being on a bicycle is the most important thing. You are a cyclist, and you should feel great about it.

WHAT CHOICE WILL YOU MAKE?

Choosing to ride a bicycle over driving a car isn't always the easiest choice, yet as more and more people do it, we show that we want and need cities and communities that are built for two wheels. The more we pedal, the easier it becomes, both for ourselves and our communities. While it would be nice to live in a world with protected bike lanes where we would never have to dodge through traffic, we can't wait for all of the right bike infrastructure to be in place; we have to ride, and we have to ride now. We have to be a part of the change that we wish to see.

Choose two wheels and enjoy the process. After all, cycling is about having fun. And who doesn't want a little more fun in their everyday lives?

Let's smile more.

Let's be happier.

Let's be healthier.

Let's ride bikes.

RESOURCES

There is a world of resources out there for whatever you want to know when it comes to bikes. The best resources are, of course, the ones closest to you—your friends who ride, your local bike shop, your local bike organization. Being a cyclist is about being a part of a community. If you have a question, don't be afraid to ask it.

ORGANIZATIONS

Whatever aspect of cycling you are looking to get into, there is probably an organization, coalition, or event out there that is happy to help you get started. Be a part of the bike revolution—get involved! From nonprofits to bike film festivals, here are a few resources to point you in the right two-wheeled direction.

ADVENTURE CYCLING ASSOCIATION →
adventurecycling.org
Established in 1973, Adventure Cycling Association's mission is to inspire and empower people to travel by bicycle. They produce cycling maps perfect for people planning a bike tour, and they publish a magazine devoted to the topic of bike travel, *Adventure Cyclist*.

ALLIANCE FOR BIKING AND
WALKING → bikewalkalliance.org
A coalition of over two hundred partners, the Alliance for Biking and Walking is dedicated to building strong communities that have safe biking and walking options.

BICYCLE FILM FESTIVAL →
bicyclefilmfestival.com

The Bicycle Film Festival is an independent festival that screens films about bike culture around the world. From Paris to Mexico City to Tokyo, the festival has been a major catalyst for the urban bike movement.

BIKE TOUR NETWORK →
biketournetwork.com

An entire network of people and organizations who love bicycle tours. The primary purpose of the network is to bring together directors, coordinators, and organizers of bicycle tours, but individuals can also use the network to find bicycle tours that they want to go on.

BLACK GIRLS DO BIKE→
blackgirlsdobike.com

Black Girls Do Bike is an organization with a mission to grow and support a community of women of color who share a passion for cycling; there are chapters around the United States.

CYCLOFEMME → **cyclofemme.com**

Are you a woman who wants to band together with other female riders? Check out Cyclofemme, a socially driven international celebration of women on bikes. Women around the world organize events for Cyclofemme day every year.

INTERNATIONAL MOUNTAIN BICYCLING ASSOCIATION → **imba.com**

Committed to creating, enhancing, and preserving great mountain biking experiences, IMBA is active in a variety of ways. You can help maintain mountain bike trails or advocate for new ones.

LEAGUE OF AMERICAN BICYCLISTS →
bikeleague.org

The League, as it's known, represents bicycles in the movement to create safer roads, stronger communities, and a bicycle-friendly America. The League is behind programs like Ride Smart, an instructional program to promote bike safety. It also offers an education program for cycle instructor certification. Their website offers an extensive list of bicycle laws, organized by state, which is helpful for finding out exactly what is and what isn't allowed in *your* state—or any state you travel to: bikeleague.org/StateBikeLaws.

PEOPLE FOR BIKES → **peopleforbikes.org**

An organization founded by bicycle industry members, People for Bikes functions both as an industry coalition and a charitable foundation. They have invested and leveraged millions of dollars in federal, state, and private funding for bicycle projects and are behind initiatives like the National Bike Challenge, running from May to September, which encourages more people to get out and ride.

RAILS-TO-TRAILS CONSERVANCY →
railstotrails.org

Founded in 1986, the Rails-to-Trails Conservancy works to transform unused rail corridors into public spaces. They run the site Trail Link (traillink.com), where you can search for trails near you, so you can easily plan a bike trip on a protected pathway.

SAFE ROUTES TO SCHOOL →
saferoutespartnership.org

Safe Routes to School is a network of hundreds of organizations, government agencies, and professional groups all working to advance safe walking and cycling to and from schools.

WOMEN'S CYCLING ASSOCIATION →
womenscyclingassociation.com

A membership organization of women cyclists and supporters committed to developing and advancing the state of women's cycling worldwide. The organization works with bicycling industry companies and organizations, as well as the media, to grow the sport of women's cycling.

WORLD BICYCLE RELIEF →
worldbicyclerelief.org

If you believe that bicycles can make a difference, then World Bicycle Relief is your organization. They provide bikes to people around the world and train local bike mechanics, all while focusing on initiatives that center on sustainable development and social enterprise.

WORLD NAKED BIKE RIDE →
worldnakedbikeride.org

Yes, this is an actual thing. There are Naked Bike Rides organized in over seventy cities in twenty different countries, so chances are if you want to bike in the nude, there's an opportunity to do so not far from you.

30 DAYS OF BIKING →
30daysofbiking.com

An initiative that runs each April, challenging participants to ride their bike every single day throughout the month.

88BIKES → 88bikes.org

Using the bike as a tool for women's empowerment, 88Bikes works to donate bicycles to girls around the world, particularly survivors of human trafficking.

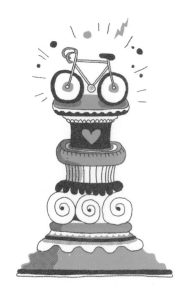

BIKE BLOGS

The Internet is full of cycling resources—and enthusiasts who love to share what's happening in the world of bikes. Here are a few of my online favorites for keeping up.

BIKE HACKS → bikehacks.com

This is the blog for anyone who loves DIY projects. The blog is full of information on fixing, tweaking, and making your bicycle the best that it can be, while also saving you some pocket change.

BIKEHUGGER → bikehugger.com

This one has been around for quite some time, and it has remained straightforward and informative. The site also publishes a monthly digital magazine.

BIKE PORTLAND → bikeportland.org

Although Portland-based and pretty focused on regional bike news and events, Bike Portland is also a go-to source for cyclists around the world interested in bike policy and beyond.

BIKE SHOP GIRL → bikeshopgirl.com

Bike Shop Girl is devoted to empowering women in cycling. Whether you're a woman who's new to cycling and looking for resources, or you want to keep up on what's happening in the world of women's professional cycling, Bike Shop Girl has it all, and the writing is smart, informative, and fun.

BIKE SNOB → bikesnobnyc.blogspot.com

Bike Snob, a well-reputed blog within the cycling world, brings a critical eye to everything from bike culture to bike policy.

COPENHAGENIZE → copenhagenize.com

Launched to document cycling culture in Copenhagen, Copenhagenize now also runs a consulting arm, working with urban planners to help "Copenhagenize" other cities around the world, showing that sustainable, functional bike infrastructure is possible anywhere.

MOMENTUM → momentummag.com

Momentum is actually a magazine, but they have a strong online profile as well, providing all kinds of resources for people interested in cycling.

THE RADAVIST → theradavist.com

The Radavist is a site devoted to the love of bicycles and getting outside. It's targeted at those who nerd out on bicycles, but even those new to the bike world can appreciate the beautiful photography, and you're sure to find some inspiration.

TOTAL WOMEN'S CYCLING → totalwomenscycling.com

A good hub for woman-focused cycling topics, from gear to training to food and nutrition.

ACKNOWLEDGMENTS

Writing a book, unlike riding a bicycle, is no simple task. This book came together thanks to the support and input of a lot of wonderful, insightful people.

Special thanks to all of the people who kindly agreed to be interviewed and who contributed to this book with their expertise: Tori Bortman, Elly Blue, David Brumsickle, Daniel Flanzig, Hannah Grant, Grant Petersen, Dan Powell, Russ Roca, Nancy Sathre-Vogel, Momoko Saunders, and Ellee Thalheimer.

Thank you to James Gulliver Hancock for his wonderful illustrations. It was lovely to work with someone as bike crazed as I am. The illustrations and text would not look the way that they do without the amazing vision of Ten Speed designer Betsy Stromberg.

To my editor, Kaitlin Ketchum: I owe you a bike tour with freshly brewed coffee every morning for believing in this project and for all of your hard work to help make it what it is.

To my mother, Britta Brones, who is always up for testing a recipe or reading through yet another one of my writing drafts, whatever the topic.

To life's best cycling partner, Luc Revel.

Of course, I never would have written a book on cycling had it not been for loving bicycles in the first place, and for that I have my father, Norman Brones, to thank. Not only for getting me on the bicycle in the first place, but also for the many adventures that we had together on our trusty blue Burley tandem. (Yes, we had matching jerseys.)

And finally, to every single person out there who rides a bike. You are the ones who keep the revolution moving forward. Keep pedaling.

INDEX

Library of Congress Cataloging-in-Publication Data

Names: Brones, Anna.
Title: Hello, bicycle : an inspired guide to the two-wheeled life / by Anna
    Brones.
Description: First Edition. | New York : Ten Speed Press, 2016 | Includes index.
Identifiers: LCCN 2015045984 (print) | LCCN 2015048609 (ebook)
Subjects: LCSH: Cycling.
Classification: LCC GV1041 .B75 2016 (print) | LCC GV1041 (ebook) | DDC
    796.6—dc23
LC record available at http://lccn.loc.gov/2015045984

Trade Paperback ISBN: 978-1-60774-883-0
eBook ISBN: 978-1-60774-884-7

Printed in China

Design by Betsy Stromberg

10 9 8 7 6 5 4 3 2 1

First Edition